Kelly Gregg MD

The Ketogenic Diet

For

Beginners

Kelly Gregg MD

THE KETOGENIC DIET FOR BEGINNERS

The Science Behind Your Diet and Why You Are Fat

Copyright 2019 by Kelly Gregg

Edition 2021

Kelly.ewriter@gmail.com

Kellygregg.com

ISBN 978-170-709-8538

KELLY GREGG MD

TABLE OF CONTENTS

CHAPTER 1

BEGINNERS

The book title is Beginner's Guide, but few among the subset of individuals buying this book are beginners. Almost all of you are buying this book because you want to lose weight. Really, you want to lose fat. You probably are content not losing much muscle mass. I am not going to judge you as to whether you need to lose weight or not. I am going to assume you have common sense and you are a rather good judge of your own body. I am also going to assume this is not your first diet. Currently, about 40% of adults in the United States are overweight or obese and this figure is increasing. Almost no one wants to be overweight or obese. Everyone uses common sense and tries to lose weight by just eating less and trying to exercise more. . This is by far the most common diet. I do not know if it is the least successful, but I think it is. The story is often that weight is initially lost, but as time goes on it's just not worth it. People just do not feel well, they have less energy, and they are hungry all the time. If it wasn't for this, the diet would work every time.

My life experience does not let me believe that this is just a massive failure of will power. These same individuals get up and go to work each day, create art, have fun, obey the law, and in general are good citizens. Why would they suddenly fail in the pursuit of weight loss? It also does not explain the epidemic of Type 2 Diabetes

(T2DM) over the last 70 years as opposed to the previous 5000. The modern diet seems to be leading us down the road of poor health. I will mention some of the reasons for this later.

Let's get going on ketosis. I am going to take you at your word that you are a beginner, hence I need to teach you a little about the lingo. In a minute we are going to go over what happens when you eat. There is a teeny bit of biochemistry involved but you will hardly notice it. First a few definitions so we are on the same page.

Diet: What you eat and when you eat. Also, what you don't eat and when you don't eat.

If you read between the lines, you may see that occasionally I am going to ask you not to eat. It will not be a big deal; in fact, you probably already do this. I just don't want you to be surprised. For you to understand the ketogenic diet, I will have to go over a few other diets.

Health: The ability to work, function in normal life, enjoy life, and be content.

This may or may not include weight loss: but I will be mentioning health, and this is what I mean.

I am going to assume you do not have any significant medical problems that would be harmful to you to be on this diet. If you are not sure, maybe you should ask someone like a health care provider. I will speak specifically about type 2 diabetes mellitus or T2DM. This book will not specifically address Type 1 or Type 3 Diabetes. Of course, I am just going to teach you the basics and you can do whatever you want to with this knowledge.

I am also going to approach this subject with the belief that your body was designed to keep you alive and functioning. It is extremely complex and has amazing recuperative powers. You can eat almost anything, and your body will process it. Today you can pick something off a tree and put it in your mouth. Next week this will be part of your toenail. You do not have to think about it, it just happens. You can also mess up this process, but your body will continue to try to adapt just to keep you going. It has mechanisms to clean up the poorly performing cellular components and keep everything in tip-top shape: if only we would not get in the way.

CHAPTER 2

<u>FOOD</u>

Your food is divided up into fats, carbohydrates, and protein. About 99% of what you eat goes into one of these categories. In this book, I am not going to care about vitamins and minerals. It is rare in this country that anyone suffers from a real vitamin deficiency disease such as rickets or scurvy. The story of vitamins and minerals is another book, full of controversy and disparaging remarks.

Let us start with fats. Fats come in two basic forms. One is a chain of carbon atoms of varying lengths which is termed a fatty acid. These usually have between 4 and 28 carbon atoms. Sometimes the carbon atoms are linked together in what is called a double bond. Saturated fatty acids mean no double bonds, unsaturated means one or more double bonds. Saturated fatty acids are more likely to be solid at normal temperatures, unsaturated more likely to be liquid. When someone says something like omega 3 fatty acid that means the double bond is at the third carbon from the omega end. An omega 6 fatty acid, double at the 6 carbon. The omega end is opposite the COOH (carboxyl) group.

For the most part this s all the biochemistry you need to know. You will hear these terms used and now at least you kind of know what they are talking about. In real life, you do not eat fatty acids.

You take three fatty acids, hook them up to a glycerol molecule, and you get a triglyceride. This is what you are eating with a piece of bacon. It is a much more compact way to store fat and does not use up as many water molecules, so this is the way nature works. When you eat fat, your stomach acids and digestive enzymes break down the triglycerides into their component fatty acid. This is what is absorbed into the body, not the triglyceride. Unlike carbohydrates and proteins, fatty acids are absorbed through the lymphatic system and dumped into the bloodstream. The other foods are absorbed and pumped right to the liver before entering the blood. That way the liver gets the first crack at the food and whatever else you may have eaten.

If it was something bad for you, the liver gets a chance to neutralize it before it goes to the rest of the body. Sometimes it does not get to it on the first pass, but the liver gets more chances as the blood circulates. Some of the lower carbon number fatty acids can also get absorbed into the blood and go right to the liver.

Now fatty acids are used in the body for energy. Most of the energy use in the body is just to keep you alive and warm. Exercise only accounts for about 20% of your energy use; the rest is the brain and other organs. Your body is very stingy about energy. Once it gets some through eating (which is the only way your body gets any energy (no photosynthesis here), it wants to keep it. So, if you eat fat, it gets turned into fatty acids, absorbed through the gut wall, recombined into triglycerides, and then gets into the bloodstream The body does not want to waste it. Certainly, some are absorbed by the cell and used right away for energy, but the rest is stored to be used later. The cell membrane converts the triglycerides back into fatty acids, and these are what are absorbed.

You already know that these fatty acids are stored in your fat cells. Fatty acids are absorbed by the fat cells and can be converted into triglyceride, which is the form of fat stored in your fat cells. Your fat cells can also go the other direction and turn triglycerides into fatty acids which are then secreted to the blood. I'll bet you can figure out what hormone controls which way the fat cell is going. Yep, it's insulin. High insulin makes the fat cell want to take up fatty acids; low insulin wants the fat cell to secrete fatty acids. Actually, the hormone glucagon may be the main driver of fatty acid release, but that only goes up if insulin goes down. If you want to lose weight you can guess which direction we want.

I must interject an additional message about fats. Much of the fat that ends up in the blood (in the form of triglycerides) comes not from the fat in your diet, but the production of fat from fructose and glucose by the liver. In other words, if you had zero fat intake, but lots of carbohydrates, you would still get fat. So, both the liver and the fat cells are in the business of making fat from sugar.

Next on the list is protein. You probably already know what protein is. It is meat. You know what it looks like and that we normally cook it. You already know your muscles are composed of protein. But wait a minute, what about these vegetarians. Well, plants contain plenty of protein. It does not look exactly like animal protein (although soy burgers are close), but it gets turned into muscle just like pork chops. Proteins are made of amino acids. There are about 20 different amino acids we use to build everything in the body. Proteins are often large molecules containing hundreds of different amino acids. All your enzymes are proteins. Your hormones sometimes contain proteins. Your heart, lungs, liver, kidneys, and skin are mainly protein. Of course, don't forget those pecs.

Proteins are usually broken down into their component amino acids and absorbed by the gut to be used by the body to make other proteins. Sometimes they are not completely broken down and actual proteins can get absorbed which sometimes causes a problem with the immune system. We need about 2-3 ounces of protein a day but often eat a lot more. Your body can use the excess for energy. The liver and kidney can take protein and turn it into glucose.

Now the king of food: Carbohydrates. Carbohydrates are sugar molecules. There are three main sugar molecules. Glucose is the primary sugar. Most of our glucose is not found free in nature, but either bound to itself in long chains or combined with another sugar molecule. The important single molecules are glucose, fructose, and galactose.

These are often bound to another sugar molecule. The important ones are sucrose, lactose, and maltose. Let's straighten these out as I find confusion reigns in this area.

Sucrose is table sugar. This is a combination of glucose and fructose. Your body easily splits these two apart and absorbs them rapidly. Remember glucose is the only sugar to which your pancreas responds with the secretion of insulin. Your pancreas is usually very good at this and can secrete lots of insulin.

Fructose is often found in fruits. This is the only single sugar of any importance found in the diet. In fruit it is combined with fiber hence it takes your gut awhile to get it absorbed, as opposed to table sugar which is rapidly split and taken up. Fruit also contains sucrose (table sugar), the combination of glucose and fructose. Some free glucose is also found in fruit. Honey is one of the few foods that contain free glucose. It is composed of about one-third fructose and one-third glucose.

Lactose is a combination of glucose and galactose. This is of importance in that some individuals lose the activity of the enzyme to split these two sugars apart as they get older and cannot digest lactose. The bacteria in the gut sure can and this leads to the production of gas and bowel discomfort. Other than this, lactose is not too important in adults. The galactose and glucose are absorbed, split apart, and the galactose converted into glucose.

Maltose is simply two glucose molecules. It ends up starch in plants is composed of long chains of glucose molecules. Your digestive tract splits off two molecules of glucose at a time which is maltose. Then it splits the maltose into individual glucose molecules which are then absorbed the normal way. In the typical American diet, we get most of our calories from starches in the form of wheat and potatoes. Just think, hamburger and French fries are mainly starch, which is saying they are mainly sugar, and that sugar is mainly glucose.

Fiber is just long chains of glucose molecules like starch, only these glucose molecules are bound together differently than starch: we do not have the enzyme to break them apart hence they are not digested and absorbed. This is why when you look at the label of the food you buy it lists total carbohydrates in grams, and under that lists dietary fiber and sugars. If you are counting total carbs, you subtract the amount of fiber from the total carbs since we are not going to digest it. Cellulose (wood) is also just a long chain of glucose molecules. We don't have that enzyme to break apart the bonds. Some animals can break apart these bonds and use cellulose for energy. I know it's really the bacteria in their stomachs that break it apart. We also have bacteria in our colon which can break down some of this fiber.

We eat sugar in the form of sucrose (table sugar), fructose (fruit sugar), lactose (milk sugar), and starch (chains of glucose). Your gut does the job of breaking this down into the individual components and we absorb them into the blood. Fructose is often bound up with fiber in fruit and it takes a little while to separate them. Starch must be broken up into individual components in the gut so that takes a little while, although not very long. Lactose is usually not a large component of the diet in adults and its claim to fame is that some people cannot digest it well.

Fiber is undigested glucose molecules that provide bulk to the stool. Now I know some of you out there claimed to be beginners, but you know that some fiber is digested by the bacteria in your large intestine. This digestion results in fatty acid production which is used locally by the cells in the colon. It also produces volatile gases which have been demonstrated by generations of teenage boys to be flammable.

A quick review of sugars shows you that the main driver of energy in the human body is going to be glucose. All the cells of the human body can use glucose to produce energy to keep you alive. Insulin facilitates the uptake of glucose by the cells of the body; however, your brain is so important it does not need insulin to use glucose. Throughout recorded history carbohydrates have been the main source of energy for the human body. One of the reasons is that they can be preserved easily to use in times of decreased food supply. It did not take our ancestors long to figure this out. You cannot store a leg of lamb very long, but you can put whole wheat kernels in a sealed clay pot and store them for years.

CHAPTER 3

<u>WE EAT</u>

Back to what happens when we eat. We are concerned with carbohydrates, and mainly glucose and fructose, whether in table sugar, fruit, or starch. Later I will talk a little about high fructose corn syrup. It won't be good.

Put food in your mouth. The first thing that happens is that you taste the food. If it tastes terrible you spit it out which for the most part is a good thing. Terrible tasting food is usually not good for you as it may be poison. Do not be afraid to spit something out. The taste of food occurs in the brain and is tied to our psychology. Sweet taste is desirable to the brain. That makes sense since the brain likes glucose. Bitter is a slight warning, but a little is OK, sour again a slight warning. Salty is something we can desire under certain circumstances. Umami is a meat-like taste that may drive us to protein. Taste is complex and another book. For our glucose attention, saliva contains an enzyme(amylase) that can break down long starch molecules in maltose. This is a two-glucose sugar molecule sugar. This is not as sweet as fructose or glucose, but it does let us know that carbs are present. The intestines then break apart these glucose molecules and you absorb simple glucose.

The stomach then sterilizes the food and begins the digestion of fat and protein. Carbs finally reach small intestines. Most of the time glucose is tied up in sucrose and starch. Sucrose is rapidly divided into glucose and fructose which are then rapidly absorbed by different mechanisms. Glucose goes into the blood then directly to the liver which then sends it to the bloodstream. The glucose is detected by the pancreas and here comes the insulin.

If you take blood out of people and put it in a tube, that's whole blood. If you spin it around without clotting and take the liquid part off, that is called plasma. If you let it clot and spin it around, now it is serum. Most of our metabolic blood tests are done on serum. Let me clear this up. It used to be those little glucose meters that used a drop of blood reported the results as blood glucose. When you went to the lab and they drew blood out of you, the report was plasma glucose. In the same sample, plasma glucose would be 10% higher than blood glucose. These days most meters just report plasma glucose, but you may need to read the fine print. Also, we in the civilized world report the results as mg/dl (milligrams per deciliter), while those barbarians in Europe use mmol/l (millimoles per liter). If you multiply mmol/l by 18, you get about the same result in mg/dl. I personally never use mmol/l because I am a patriotic American.

Back to the liver. The liver also stores glycogen. Glycogen is like animal starch. It is a highly branched string of glucose molecules the liver can break apart one glucose molecule at a time. The liver makes sure the brain is happy by keeping the glucose level stable by either releasing glucose from glycogen or making glucose out of protein. Remember you have lots of protein, even more than fat. The liver is always adding or subtracting from its glycogen supply.

Your body is stingy about glucose. Once the plasma glucose level gets around 200 mg/dl, glucose begins to be lost in the urine. Your body does not like that, so it tries to save the glucose energy. It does this by secreting insulin which hastens the absorption of glucose by the cells of the body, especially the muscle cells. The higher the plasma sugar, the more insulin is secreted. It also tries to save energy by storing it in fat cells. Glucose goes into the fat cell, is converted to fatty acids, and then saved as triglycerides. The higher the insulin, the more this process takes place. If you happen to have low insulin, this process goes in the other direction, however, once the glucose is converted to fatty acids by the fat cells, it does not go back to glucose. Fatty acids are released instead. High levels of glucose are directly toxic to cells in the body, so if it gets too high, getting rid of it in the urine is the last resort. Your body is going to keep absorbing it as long as you keep eating it.

For every glucose molecule in table sugar, there is a fructose molecule. Fructose does not stimulate insulin production and insulin does not enhance the absorption of fructose. It is still able to be absorbed by cells and used for energy, just not nearly as well as glucose. Virtually all metabolism of fructose takes place in the liver. A little is used by the sperm for energy. When it hits the liver, it is used to make glycogen. It also is converted into fatty acids and triglycerides. It takes a while for the liver to do this, so the fructose wanders around in your bloodstream a while. Later I'll tell you why you don't want this.

Let us be clear. You eat sucrose (table sugar) and get glucose and just as much fructose. The glucose gets gobbled up by the tissue to be used as energy. The fructose gets turned into glucose and made into glycogen by the liver, it also turns a lot of the fructose into fatty acids and hence to triglycerides just like the fat cells. These triglycerides are not saved in the liver but sent into blood bonded to what are called lipoproteins, which then carry them around to be used or saved in the fat cells along with the glucose derived triglyceride. The lipoproteins carry cholesterol, a fat, in addition to the triglycerides.

The brain has a strange relationship with fructose. It does not use it for energy, but rather uses up energy metabolizing fructose. Recently we figured out that when your glucose levels get too high, the brain converts glucose into fructose. Remember a couple of things. Your brain does not need insulin to absorb glucose; hence controlling the insulin does not control the absorption. Elevated glucose levels are toxic to cells; even brain cells (maybe especially brain cells). If your glucose levels are elevated, lowering the insulin level does not keep the brain from absorbing it. The brain may be protecting itself from the elevated glucose levels by converting some of it to fructose. You do not want a lot of fructose floating around in your brain either.

Later when I talk about T2DM we will also talk about dementia. Your body is amazingly complex, and we just don't understand it completely. I am starting you out as a beginner. You will not be one when we finish. Do not worry. Even if you are only barely paying attention and only have a sliver of motivation, I will get you to lose fat. You have already failed a diet that theoretically should work every time, which is to just eat less. That did not work. I could just make this a book of one page and just say "Eat this and don't eat this". But that would probably fail also. I am going to do my best to get you to understand the ketogenic diet to lose weight. You will also understand why this should work every time. We know that this does not work every time, but there is a much greater chance you will lose weight on this diet than other weight loss diets.

My life experience tells me that if you know why you are doing something, and if it is of great advantage to you to do this, you are more likely to do it. You must trust me a little bit. I am teaching various concepts and in a certain order such that at the end of the book you will understand it better. I am not your doctor or health care provider, but I am your teacher. As you continue reading, you may very well know more about this subject than most health care providers and make your own informed decisions. Stay with me and fight through a little more science.

We ate protein and absorbed the amino acids. There is not a lot of disease related to that. This is related to inflammation, gut bacteria, and absorption, but that is a different book.

We ate fat and absorbed the fatty acids. Not a lot of disease related to that. All fats are not the same. This is a different chapter.

We ate carbohydrates and absorbed sugar. A lot of disease related to this and here is our pathway. The glucose has arrived, and the pancreas is pumping out insulin. We are trying to keep the level from getting too high by getting the muscles to absorb it, getting the fat cells to absorb it, converting it to fructose in the brain, and, if necessary, sending it out in the urine. If your pancreas is normal, it can make plenty of insulin. Eventually, if we stop eating and the glucose level returns to normal. We can ask what is normal? That can change throughout your life.

There is a metabolic and glucose set point in your body. Most people do not pay much attention to how much or what they eat. They eat when they are hungry and stop when they are full. Amazingly enough, this works quite well. Most can keep their weight within a few pounds for years with little effort. As time goes on, we may notice a pound or two of weight gain a year. If our life changes dramatically the weight gain or loss may change more rapidly. But usually, we are minding our own business and suddenly realize after twenty or thirty years that none of our clothes fit. Apparently, our setpoint has changed. What changes that setpoint is more complicated and is related to age, activity, health, diet, and psychology. It does not matter. Here we are and we don't like it.

Your setpoint for the glucose level may change as you age. I mean like in 20 – 30 years. I am a little more confident that this is related to your diet. In most people, the problem is not the pancreas not putting out enough insulin, it's the opposite. It's just the insulin isn't having the same effect. There is nothing wrong with the insulin, but rather the receptors on the cells don't seem to be using it as well. Let's give two examples that we already know about.

Your body changes as time goes on, your diet changes, or your activities change. If you start lifting weights, you may develop more lean body mass (muscles). You expect that to happen. You have induced certain biochemical processes in the muscle cells to use energy more efficiently or grow and repair more rapidly or operate better despite a lower oxygen supply or just look better. You did this by inducing certain metabolic processes that required enzymes or transport proteins. In other words, the DNA in the cells started replicating and producing more RNA that coded for more proteins that cause increased absorption of amino acids that cause the ribosomes to make more molecules of various enzymes or receptors, that caused, well lots of things.

This does not happen overnight. It may take years to induce this activity to its full effect. The same can happen in reverse if you stop lifting weights. This induction of processes happens all over the body: Sometimes a little faster in certain cells, sometimes very slowly in certain cells.

Your body cells also have receptors for insulin on the surface of the cell. When stimulated by insulin it activates the process to absorb glucose (and by the way also amino acids) into the cell thus lowering the amount of glucose in the blood. As we age, the amount of glucose in the blood varies. If you are someone eating a lot of glucose, you will secrete more insulin. If you eat often, you will have more episodes of insulin secretion. Do this for 30 years. Over that time your muscle cells did not have to work that hard-to-get glucose. There was always plenty around at a high level and the cell did not have to work that hard to get it. Do you think that maybe you would induce the cell not to make as many insulin receptors?

Your body is highly adaptive. It will not waste energy making a lot of insulin receptors if it does not need a lot of receptors to get glucose. Over the years we know what happens. You need fewer receptors to get the job done. If we were always low on glucose, your body would make more receptors to suck out the glucose as fast as it can. High levels of glucose give lower numbers of receptors and no hurry to get the glucose sucked out, there is always plenty around. Of course, your pancreas is not quite as smart, so it keeps pumping out a little more insulin to get that glucose down as it does not seem to be dropping as fast as it used to. Also, the glucose receptors in the pancreas are always being exposed to a high level of glucose so they are not quite as sensitive to the blood level. The set point of the glucose level begins creeping up.

After a while, you figure out what we get. The resting glucose level has gone up; however, the insulin level has also gone up. Eventually, we get what is called insulin resistance. Despite plenty of good insulin around, the blood level of glucose is higher.

In the meantime, let us see what those fat cells have been doing all these years. Insulin stimulates the fat cells to take up glucose and store it as fat. After all, the insulin levels would not be elevated unless the glucose level was elevated, and we want to save that energy. Similarly, if the insulin levels are low, that means the glucose level is low, and now we need to pump out fatty acids to give the body enough energy. The fat cells just care about insulin levels. In Type 1 diabetes, there is not enough insulin despite high glucose levels; hence the fat cells are not storing glucose. You get skinny children with high glucose levels.

If we have high insulin levels, guess what we are inducing. It is complicated to convert glucose into triglycerides and requires lots of different proteins and enzymes. If you have chronically elevated insulin levels, your fat DNA finally produces enough biochemical infrastructures that you get rather good at changing glucose into fat. This takes years to finally get up to speed, but once there it works great.

At the same time, you have not been going the other way that often. You have not induced the conversion of triglycerides to fatty acids, so your fat stores are slowly getting bigger and bigger as if we had not already noticed that. There is some hope. It is not quite as complicated to convert triglycerides to fat and does not take quite as long to induce. Although this process may not have been used for a while, it is more important to get energy out when needed than to add to an already large supply of stores. Hence your body is smart enough that this process can be induced faster if needed. And this is exactly what we want for weight loss.

CHAPTER 4

<u>WE STOP EATING</u>

Now you know what happens when you eat carbs. Mainly, the glucose level goes up. The pancreas can regulate the amount of insulin such that within a couple of hours after finishing the meal, the glucose level is almost back to normal with none lost out the urine. We can do a test in which you drink 75 grams of a glucose solution, and we measure your plasma level two hours later. If it is under 140 mg/dl, you pass. It ends up that the glucose tolerance test may be the first metabolic abnormality noted in those who are developing a resistance to insulin. It is positive long before the fasting glucose level becomes abnormal.

If you are normal, the glucose level becomes normal and the insulin level drops to its baseline value. This value should be low enough that little glucose is being converted into fat. Both glucose going to fat and fatty acids coming out of fat cells never goes to completely zero. There is always a little going in each direction and the amount is dictated by insulin.

You have stopped eating, but your body continues to use energy to keep you alive. Despite not having any input, your liver keeps the glucose level stable by digesting the glycogen stored there. This is prompted by the hormone glucagon which is also secreted by the pancreas. Glucagon is secreted by the alpha cells in the pancreas; insulin is secreted by the beta cells, Yin and Yang. If insulin secretion increases, glucagon levels decrease. If insulin goes down, glucagon goes up. The increase in glucagon increases the liver's conversion of glycogen to glucose release.

There are about 100 grams of glucose stored in the liver in the form of glycogen which can keep your brain happy about a day. Remember your brain needs glucose to be happy and does not need insulin to get it. So, the insulin level stays low and the liver keeps adding glucose to the blood. Your skeletal muscles also store glycogen. It stores about four times as much as the liver. This will enable your muscles to work at an endurance exercise for 2-3 hours. It also saves the blood glucose allowing your brain to use it instead of wasting it on skeletal exercise. The glucose in your skeletal muscles is not released to the blood. Glucose goes in, makes glycogen, which is broken down for use in the muscle, but none of the glucose comes back out.

Things are stable for now, but you can see that this cannot go on forever or we will run out of glucose. It's not that we eventually may not be able to walk, but we sure want to continue thinking. Since the insulin is now low, your glucagon level is high, and it stimulates your fat cells to begin sending fatty acids out of the cell instead of taking glucose into the cell and converting it into fatty acids.

Fatty acids are a great source of energy. One gram of glucose is equivalent to 4 calories. A calorie is a measurement of energy. One gram of fat gives us 9 calories. We have lots of potential energy available and the fat cells are putting these out into the blood. Almost all the cells in your body enjoy using fatty acids and will gladly take them into the cell. No insulin needed. This keeps us chugging along with no difficulty. Unfortunately, your pesky brain does not use fatty acids for energy. The clock is still ticking, and the glucose level is still slowly dropping, despite everybody except your brain using fatty acids. (red blood cells also need glucose but that usually is not an issue)

Your liver (and your kidneys) starts making glucose from protein. Like most other metabolic processes, there is always a little of this going on all the time. With the drop in the glucose levels glucagon, adrenaline, cortisol, and growth hormone all start stimulating the liver to begin making glucose.

Now we have glucose slowly going down, fatty acids going up, glucagon is stimulating the release of glycogen glucose in the liver, muscles using up their glycogen and starting to use fatty acids, and the liver starting to make new glucose from protein. You can see it's somewhat of a race to keep enough glucose around to feed the brain. Now we get a new player in the game. As the fatty acid level begins rising and new glucose is being produced, a product of this metabolism in the liver is the production of ketone bodies.

A ketone body can be thought of as a metabolic product of fatty acid metabolism. These are smaller molecules than fatty acids and can be used by most cells in the body. Most importantly, the brain can use ketones instead of glucose for energy. Now we have ketone bodies starting up also, so our brain is happy again. It is rare that anyone will pass out if they don't eat for a day and the brain quits working well. Almost all the time the brand-new glucose, the ketone bodies, and the glycogen glucose will be sufficient to power our brains.

Finally, we are in a stable situation. Now what? You know, if we wanted to lose fat, why do anything. Our brain is happy. The fat cells are slowly getting smaller. It seems we have reached our goal. The problem is most people get hungry and start the whole cycle all over again. It seems like we are back where we started and, other than the reduced calorie diet which does not seem to work very well. We are going to have to do something different. Now we are going to have to talk about diets. After all, this is a diet book.

CHAPTER 5

PAST DIETS

The concept of the best diet has only been an issue in the last hundred years or so. To understand previous diets, we can go back a few thousand years when there is a written history. The Egyptians have a good chronology and historical record that goes back about five thousand years ago. They also have pictures. The Bible has written history going back about that same time frame. About 2500 years ago several cultures in various parts of the world began recording history. The dietary history is skewed as, unless you had an abundance of food, you did not have a civilization or city. In order to have science and government, you must have enough extra food to feed these people in the city. Hence when you look back, it appears there was plenty of food available over the last few thousand years.

Mankind was not in a state of near starvation and in fact, famines appeared to be rare.   Decreased food supply was usually related to war or other government events. This makes some sense as if you were in a location in the world and there was not enough food, you went somewhere else. There are certainly records of commerce several thousand years ago where food was sold. This is important as a farmer has the motivation to grow more food than he needs and be able to trade this extra food for something else. Therefore, capitalism generally results in plentiful food.

Food appeared to be much more regional before the advent of effective food storage. Food has been dried and salted for several thousand years. To survive in most areas, you must preserve food. Crops and fruits are only ripe certain times of the year. Even keeping animals requires that fodder must be available during the winter. Even if you lived by the ocean there was a seasonal aspect to the availability of fresh food. The easiest types of food to store are starches. Grains, root vegetables, tubers, pumpkins, and squash can be kept in the appropriate environment for months. Dried fruit has long been stored for times of scarcity.

As you can imagine, meat and fats are more difficult to store for several months. It does seem that mankind enjoyed eating fat. Of course, this is the most difficult type of food to preserve. Hence, during lean times like winter or among the poorer folk, the diet was heavy on carbohydrates. Grains do provide some protein and fat and are quite amenable to long term storage. Grain can also be fed to animals during the winter and hence enable protein storage on the hoof. For the most part in the last few thousand years, although there appeared to be plenty of food, the diet of most people during scarcity was heavy on carbohydrates. This was not a low carbohydrate diet, there was plenty of food; then how come there was not an obesity epidemic?

Your body can adapt to almost any diet and keep you healthy. Remember my working definition of health is to able to work, function in normal life, enjoy life, and be content. It appears that throughout written history your body has been able to keep you healthy. Is it just me or does it appear that during the last 50 years it hasn't been able to accomplish that goal as well?

The days of our years are threescore and ten; and if by reason of strength they be fourscore years, yet is their strength labour and sorrow: for it is soon cut off and we fly away.

 Psalm 90:10

This verse was written about 3400 years ago

Life expectancy for men aged 50 years is 25.5 years

This statistic was written in 2018

The point is our body worked great as far as diet is concerned for recorded history. It can adapt to low carbohydrate, high carbohydrate, low protein, high protein, high calorie, low calorie, fasting, and even starvation to keep you alive and healthy. What is different with the modern diet?

We tend to discount those who lived long ago as though they were not nearly as smart as we are now. We change our diets based on the current "scientific thought". We conveniently forget how often this has been wrong. We discount a thousand years of trial and error, proving what works over the long haul. What do we learn from history and diet? It was probably not low carbohydrate. It was probably not based on recurrent episodes of starvation. It was primarily based on what was available and what was able to be stored.

For the most part, there was probably a lot of food. It also appeared that people like variety in their diet and went through a lot of trouble getting different spices, growing different crops, and getting different foods from different lands. Sweets were desired and this mainly revolved around fruits where the sugars were bound to fiber. Honey was available and highly desirable, both as a preservative and sweetener. Nobody was eating table sugar.

In general, people ate during the daytime. It was difficult to eat at night and artificial light was a wasteful use of energy. People ate a little while after the sun came up and a little while before the sun went down. The concept of a midday meal started becoming popular a few hundred years ago. It became popular the last couple hundred years when artificial light allowed the last meal of the day to be later and extended the time between breakfast and dinner. I think the concept of food between breakfast and lunch, between lunch and dinner, between dinner and sleep, is a more recent practice.

CHAPTER 6

MODERN DIETS

We have already mentioned the normal diet. People eat until they are full. They then eat again when hungry and convenient. Believe it or not, this works most of the time. Your body has a hormone (leptin) that makes you feel full. Some people can eat an additional thin mint even though their body is screaming at them that they are full. If you start exercising, your body will make you a little hungrier. If you are sedentary, you are not quite as hungry. People certainly can eat when not hungry and not stop eating when they are full, but for most of their life, this diet seems to work.

Most everyone in this country has a basic knowledge of nutrition. Even a teenager knows it is probably not a great idea to eat cherry pie for every meal. Most know they need to eat a little variety. Most know if they are getting fat then they probably are not eating correctly. Let us not discount the primary motivation for most people ages 15-30 to not get fat: they wish to increase their ability to attract the opposite sex. Of course, this motivation appears to decrease after being married for twenty years, right around the time most people are getting fat.

This technique appears to be failing in modern times. Obesity is becoming quite a problem, and along with this Type 2 Diabetes (T2DM). There are many factors why obesity is a problem now and not over the previous 5000 years. We can blame the availability of food 24 hours a day, or the increase in processed food, or the effectiveness of advertising, or the increased use of table sugar, or the increased use of modern flour, or the rising standard of living and increase in dining out. I don't think we can particularly blame decreased exercise. Exercise is not a primary determinant of fat, diet is.

In history, there have always been a few fat people. These people were usually well off and ate lots of food. During the 1800s and early 1900s, there was increased interest in the diet of isolated peoples around the world. African natives, remote islanders, Inuit: All were examined, and the story is always the same. Once they started eating a Western diet with flour, sugar, molasses, they all started getting fat and developing western diseases. This was regardless of their previous diet. Even those who had a higher carbohydrate diet changed with the Western diet. Although the higher carbohydrate diet was somewhat responsible, it also appears that processed food (table sugar, milled grains) had an additional effect.

In 1700 the average sugar consumption in America was 1 tsp a day, in 1800 it was 4 tsp a day, in 1900 it was 28 tsp a day, and in 2009 about 50% of Americans consumed 52 teaspoons a day of sucrose. I think we can see part of the problem. Average wheat consumption has risen 25% in the last 40 years. We all agree we are eating more sugar and wheat. Remember wheat is mainly starch which is mainly glucose.

We already know from the last chapter what happens when we eat a lot of glucose. Our brain is happy, and our fat cells are busy. So how come we eat so much? This is a difficult question. We seem to be driven to eat sweets. Before modern civilization (before 1700), sweets were hard to come by. Mainly they occurred in fruits. Our average fructose intake used to be about 20 grams a day. Remember fruits only used to be eaten a few months a year when the fruit was ripe. Also, fructose was bound with fiber and hence took a little while to be absorbed. Now we are up to 80grams a day of fructose (Dept of Agriculture estimate food disappearance data). There is more fruit eaten as now we can eat it every day of the year if we want and remember half of sucrose is fructose. Now we have the new heroin, high fructose corn syrup (HFCS). I'll discuss that in a minute.

I think it is fair to say that now we can eat sugar whenever we want, be it fructose, sucrose, or even lactose. Our brain still is wired to seek sweets as this a ready and easy supply of calories and our liver and fat cells are set up to convert this into fat for later use in case we run out of food. It is even more complicated. When artificial sweeteners (very low calorie) came onto the market, they were touted as a cure for obesity. All you had to do was keep eating the same diet and substitute artificial sugar for the real thing. This was mainly true with soda pop. If you drank one can of pop a day, just switch to diet pop and you must lose weight. After all, it is like a reduced calorie diet. Eat fewer calories and you have to lose weight. Many studies have been done. It just does not work.

Theories abound as to why it does not work; most revolve around the brain and the desire for sweetness. Artificial sweeteners are more potent than sugar and seem to drive a desire for sugar. Many of you have tried to lay off sugar for a while and most noticed that when they go back to eating sugar, things taste sweeter. It is as if you were inducing the number of sweet taste buds since the amount of sugar was down. Say you do the opposite and use very sweet artificial sweeteners; you may induce the opposite, so it requires more sweet to give the brain the same satisfaction. People who use artificial sweeteners seem to have a craving for sweetness. You can drink 10 cans of diet Coke a day and still, this is not enough. By the way, in most people this is too much.

So, our modern diet has food available 24 hours a day, has multiple choices for almost any food, is replete with various forms of desserts and pastry items, is affordable, and is advertised on TV throughout the day and night. Do not underestimate the power of modern advertising. This is a science unto itself.

Now you may be saying "I give up. I am no match for the forces arrayed against me". Normally I would agree with you, but fortunately, we have instinctive drives so that we are going to keep trying to survive. Good thing one of our strongest drives is the sex drive. We simply do not want to look obese in this society because it may decrease our chance of reproduction.

This works well in younger folks. As we get older, we want to work. This may motivate us to eat better so we are not as tired, feel better, and are more productive. Then we want to think. Most are more worried about getting dementia than dying. This may primarily be a dietary issue. Finally, we want to live. Men especially want to be healthy till they die. And they are in no hurry to die. Innately we believe that some combination of lifestyle, exercise, and diet may be the key to living longer. This comes as a result of common senses, not experimental evidence.

This is a book about the ketogenic diet and losing weight, not particularly about psychology or religion. I will convince you of the best method for you to lose fat. You will understand why it works. I will compare this to the other weight loss diets.

We must face the fact that you really cannot be on a weight loss diet forever. I have run across many people who always seem to be on a diet. Obviously, it is not working well. If your weight loss diet is working, you will get to the weight you have determined to be optimal for you. I hope you are practical in this determination. Your ideal weight is probably not the weight you were when you were 18. I would be remiss if we did not discuss what you are going to do when you achieve this ideal weight. You will have to be on a long-term maintenance diet, one not designed to be a weight loss diet. We will discuss that at the end.

CHAPTER 7

METABOLIC STATES

Remember the definition of diet I am using. A diet is what you eat and when you eat. Also, it is when you don't eat. Different diets produce different metabolic states which are different biochemical states in your body.

We will start with history. For most of recorded history, man ate twice a day in accordance with the rhythm of the sun. Probably no lunch. No midnight snack. No eating between commercials on TV. Most of the time there was at least 12 hours between the last meal of the day and the first of the next day. We know what happens when you eat unless you skipped that chapter. You get a rise in the insulin level which returns to normal 2-3 hours later. Your insulin receptors are exposed to insulin for a couple of hours, your fat cells are exposed to insulin for a couple of hours, and glucagon is then released for a few hours until we eat again. During those times between eating, the insulin is low, glycogen is being metabolized to maintain glucose levels, the liver is starting to make glucose from protein, and fatty acids are being released from the fat cells. Not many ketones are being created unless this time frame is extended. You start eating again 6-8 hours later and the cycle repeats.

You have a total time of exposure to elevated insulin of about 4-6 hours in a 24-hour period. You also have a 12 hour fast every day. During that fasting time, you are again in a different metabolic state. You now are starting to make a few ketones. You are changing your hormonal production as your body is preparing you for not eating. Although your body is very adaptive, it does not know when you will eat again. There is a metabolic state that exists when fasting that changes your entire hormonal milieu. At the 12-hour mark, this metabolic state is getting up-regulated. Then we eat again and the cycle repeats.

I believe some version of this metabolic state has been the rule for the majority of history. Artificial lighting changed this pattern for everyone. In fact, I believe you would be hard-pressed to find many people in America who would fit into this metabolic state.

SPOILER ALERT: Before the end of this book, I am going to talk you into the daily 12 hours fast. Later you will learn about a bunch of things that happen to your benefit if you just stop eating for a while.

Every time you eat carbs, even one bonbon, your insulin level pops up. It then eventually goes back down, but you can see that eating numerous times during the day leads to an almost continuous exposure to insulin during that time. You can guess what continuous exposure leads to.

So now you know about the historical metabolic state and the modern metabolic state. You have an idea as to what is going on in your body regarding diet. You now should know you need insulin to survive, but insulin exposure all the time is not a good idea. Since this is a fat loss book, we will look at the metabolic states of a few more diets.

What happens metabolically with the reduced calorie diet? You are going along in life eating when you are hungry and not eating when you are not. This has worked well but eventually; you want to lose a little fat. You decide to decrease the number of calories. No big change in what happens when you eat; you just don't eat as much. Still with the same number of meals and about the same amount of total insulin secreted. What you have missed is the secretion of leptin. Leptin is a hormone secreted primarily by the fat cells and helps regulate energy balance by inhibiting hunger. Remember you have a set energy balance level. Therefore, most of the time you do not have to pay much attention to how much you eat and still have an almost constant weight. When you take in fewer calories, your leptin levels decrease, and you get hungry. Not only that, but you also get cranky, depressed, and fatigued. One way your body will compensate for fewer calories is to lower the metabolic rate. So, when you just cut back on calories, your energy decreases.

Now you are going to say that you just need to lower your energy balance set point. I agree but how to do that? Just like if this thing worked so well, how come I slowly gained weight over the years? Is it because I just do not exercise as much? You may not exercise as much but that's not the reason. How come my body did not just reduce my eating when I reduced my exercise?

The problem is insulin. As you can see, this book is starting to rotate around insulin, and insulin rotates around carbohydrates. Fat rotates around insulin and leptin rotates around fat cells. OK, what is going on? I just told you that for most of human history, carbohydrates have been the mainstay of the diet. For most of human history, there has been plenty of food around.   For most of human history, 40% of us have not been overweight. Why is something screwed up with insulin in the last 70 or so years? I will give you a hint. It's your diet.

Back to the reduced calorie diet. It makes you hungry. It decreases your leptin which makes you depressed. It also decreases your active thyroid hormone which makes you feel that you have less energy and not only that, but your decreased metabolic state also makes it harder to lose weight. I am not saying it can never work, but by far it is the most failed diet of modern times. I say modern times because for most history, getting on a diet to lose weight was unheard of. Now you can't walk down the street without tripping over a diet book.

I will mention this diet is passing as a warning; the famous low- fat diet. This was quite popular 20-50 years ago when cholesterol was all the rage. The medical profession started measuring cholesterol and decided that elevated cholesterol was the curse of man that caused cardiovascular disease. Now I agree cardiovascular disease is a bad thing. Certainly, elevated cholesterol (whatever that number may really be) is a factor in heart disease. There are several other factors including genetics, but cholesterol became easily measured hence, we decided that we must treat it.

Nowadays we have numerous effective medications that will definitely lower your cholesterol. I do not know if it will prevent cardiovascular disease, but there seems to be little doubt that if you get a heart attack, taking statins after this will prolong your life; Maybe despite whether it lowers your cholesterol or not. Will taking statins prevent a heart attack from occurring in the first place? Not sure of the risk-benefit.

Anyway, there were not a lot of cholesterol-lowering medications back then, so the medical profession decided to recommend a low-fat diet. By now you understand what that means. Low fat means higher protein and carbohydrates. The low-fat diet did not advise high protein, so everyone ended up with a high carbohydrate diet. Even you as a beginner now know that high carbs equals high glucose burden equals elevated insulin equals fat cells getting bigger equals 20-30 years later Type 2 Diabetes (T2DM) I'll talk about that later but let me say T2DM is worse than a little elevated cholesterol. The low-fat diet lowered the cholesterol maybe 10-20%. Most of the cholesterol in your body is made by you.

This is a warning as this diet probably did more harm than good. Yet it was promoted by all the dietitians and cardiac physicians. They were wrong. Now we have the cure-all ketogenic diet. I do believe this is better for weight loss. I don't believe you should be on it for the rest of your life. But I have been wrong before and will probably be wrong again. I hope by the end of this book you can evaluate any diet and make a reasonable decision. The medical profession should be honored, but they are not infallible. I am not giving you medical advice, but my personal opinion is that for most people the low-fat diet is not a good diet.

CHAPTER 8

T2DM and AGEs

Believe it or not, now is the time to talk about diabetes. I know you are waiting around for the ketogenic diet, and I will get to that. You have to trust me this comes first. There may be a few people who bought this book because they have T2DM. Others got the book because they did not want to get T2DM.

I have tried many times to get people to quit smoking. I have not been very successful, with one exception. I can get them to quit smoking after they have their first heart attack.

I have tried many years to get people to eat right and lose weight. I am much more successful after their doctor tells them they have diabetes or now, pre-diabetes. One of the primary risks of T2DM, other than cardiovascular disease, is dementia. People are more afraid of that then a heart attack. T2DM is a great risk factor for Alzheimer's. Now I can get your attention.

You already know the deal. Too much sucrose and other carbs, eating too often, continuous insulin elevation, finally you start to get used to the high insulin levels and the receptors don't work so well. The insulin is still working great in your fat cells and is pushing that glucose in to be converted to fat. Finally, the blood sugar states to rise. Before that happened, we could have done a glucose tolerance test and measured either the actual insulin or the blood sugar and see that there was an abnormality. By the time your pancreas is not getting your blood sugar down to a normal baseline, you essentially have T2DM. T2DM is caused by insulin resistance. This causes an elevation of not only insulin but also blood sugar; a metabolic state that should not exist.

If you are obese, you probably have some insulin resistance. You may not have T2DM yet, but it is on the horizon. You may want to think about doing something.

Before that I must explain Advanced Glycation End Products or what we call AGEs. I never heard much about them till a few years ago, now I think this is one of the main drivers of the complications of diabetes.

The easiest way to explain them is to use the Hemoglobin A1c test. Many of you already know what this test is designed to do. The A1c test can tell us what your average blood sugar was over the past three months. This is a great test. We have decreed that if your A1c is less than 5.7, you do not have diabetes, between 5.7 and 6.4, and then you have prediabetes. At 6.5 or greater, maybe you have diabetes (not yet an official diagnostic criteria)

Glycation is the covalent (chemical) bonding of a sugar molecule (glucose and fructose mainly) to a protein or fat without the assistance of an enzyme. It turns out fructose has ten times the glycation activity as glucose. Now you have millions of bonds forming or breaking apart every second in the cells of your body.

Most all of these bond formations are controlled by enzymes. In glycation, there is no real control.

The glucose can bind in numerous sites of a protein resulting in the protein not fitting correctly in a receptor (abnormal folding of a protein). The protein could not work as well or not work at all. Possibly the glycation made no difference. Another problem is that once the protein is abnormal, you may not be able to digest it as well. Remember we have enzymes to build protein out of amino acids, and enzymes designed to cut them apart in certain places. We may not be able to get rid of some of these abnormal proteins.

A1c represents the amount of glucose that has been bound to the hemoglobin in the red blood cells. It is essentially an AGE. These cells live about 120 days. Once the glucose has been glycated, it does not deglycate. If you do the math and I have not, the A1c test is a picture of the average amount of glucose this red blood cell has been exposed to over the last 90 days.

Now this red blood cell is going to get recycled and it only lived about 120 days, but some cells in your body last longer than that. They have the same problem, getting rid of these abnormal glycated proteins. There is a process called autophagy that can manage to clean up these AGEs, but even that process can be overwhelmed. Guess what overwhelms it, high levels of glucose. Alzheimer's is an accumulation of abnormal protein in the brain eventually resulting in plaques. It may be related to a lifetime of AGE accumulation. There is no doubt an elevated glucose level increases AGEs. There is no doubt that T2DM increases the risk of Alzheimer's, also Parkinson's.

Apparently, it is possible to overwhelm autophagy. Once the plaque forms, it cannot be removed. Treatment is going to involve diagnosing the risk early on and doing something about it. If there was only some way to activate autophagy earlier in life. That would be a great deal since we also believe AGEs are one of the main causes of aging throughout the body. It would be amazing if your body was created to stimulate autophagy to possibly delay some of these aging symptoms. I guess there is just nothing to be done.

We have insulin resistance, we are obese, and we have elevated blood sugar, what can we do? We need to ameliorate insulin resistance. This took years to develop and exposure to a lot of glucose. I think we know what must be done. We must lower carbohydrates in our diet. We must go on some type of low carbohydrate diet. At this point, you do not get a choice. Your T2DM is going to slowly progress. We have lots of medications that may get your glucose levels lower, but the normal course of events is that as time goes on, we must keep adding additional medications to keep keeping it lower. I say lower because most of the time it is still not normal. We still have not affected your insulin resistance.

Lowering your blood sugar with medication does not usually get rid of fat. Exercising more does not fix you. The only treatment that gives you a chance is dietary. I can get you to stop smoking after a heart attack; this is the metabolic equivalent of a heart attack. Change your ways or bad things will happen. Treating T2DM costs a lot of money, is very inconvenient, makes you go to the doctor all the time, and you just aren't participating in my definition of health.

I want you to do something cheap, effective, productive, and may lead you to health.

If you bought this book just to lose a little fat, we will do this. You will lose weight with a ketogenic diet. You cannot be on this for the rest of your life and if you go back to your normal diet the fat may reappear, but you will and can lose it.

If you have T2DM it's a different story. You can never go back to your previous diet. Fat loss will not cure you. You cannot be on a continuous ketogenic diet for years. You must change your diet permanently to some version of a low carb diet to help manage your T2DM. You have no choice.

CHAPTER 9

AUTOPHAGY

We are so close to talking about ketogenesis, but I realize I left you hanging in the last chapter. You may be a beginner, but now you get a postgraduate course. Some of you may not understand the next few paragraphs, but the next time you hear them they will sound familiar.

Now I'm no dummy, at least by the official medical definition, but I had not heard of this until a few years ago. Now I can't live without it. Of course, no one can, but it did make a lot of things make sense. Autophagy is pronounced auto-fay-gee, at least by all patriotic Americans. It is a lysosome -dependent homeostatic process in which organelles or proteins are degraded and recycled into energy. DO NOT FREAK OUT. You will only be embarrassing yourself. I will explain.

The cells in your body contain little cystic structures called lysosomes. Inside these cysts are acids and digestive enzymes. You must be careful not to let any of these contents leak out or you will start digesting the whole cell. There may be quite a few of these in a cell. Homeostasis is the process of doing whatever it takes to stay alive. There are all kinds of homeostatic mechanisms in a cell from gathering energy to building proteins to translating DNA. Autophagy is one of these processes that are required for cell survival.

There are all kinds of proteins and other structures in your cells that may not be working very well. Sometimes the little organs in the cell wear out like the mitochondria. Nothing is perfect and sometimes the DNA transcription messes up a little and the wrong amino acid gets put in a protein. The protein may still work fine, just not quite as well as the original. Sometimes the DNA itself gets messed up and starts producing abnormal protein. This can screw things up. Sometimes we call that cancer.

Your body is smart. There is a complex mechanism whereby these abnormal structures can be identified, tagged, and transported to one of these lysosomes. When it gets there, the protein or structure is dissolved down to its constituent units like amino acids or fatty acids or sugars. These then can be used to make new proteins or used as energy. This whole process is called autophagy.

You can see that if you had a cell that lived years, it would accumulate a lot of these less than ideal structures and would need to be cleaned out occasionally. Some of this trash is the AGEs we talked about earlier. Autophagy is something we like. We should encourage this activity. You can see why this is referred to as an anti-aging process as aging is the accumulation of old stuff in the cell. We want new stuff in the cell and since the cell can make all the stuff, why isn't it all new stuff. Well maybe it was designed to be all new stuff, but that darn autophagy isn't keeping up to speed.

Like a lot of other processes we have discussed, autophagy can be induced. The more it is used the more activity occurs and the greater the maximum activity can be. As you can see, autophagy requires hundreds of proteins, all these must be coded from DNA and replicated in the cells. Inducing autophagy means increasing a lot of different proteins and enzymes and is going to take some time, like years. Regardless, like the other homeostatic process, there is always a little going on. We want a lot going on. So, the question is "What stimulates autophagy?".

Autophagy is stimulated by Intermittent Metabolic Stress. This makes sense when you think about it. When the cell is under stress, you want it to work as efficiently as possible. You do not want any freeloaders hanging around. In fact, we want to use those freeloaders as parts to make new proteins or turn them into energy to make these new proteins work. Autophagy does not get rid of old cells, it does whatever it takes to keep these old cells alive by getting rid of the trash and encouraging brand new proteins. It wants to make your cells young again.

OK, how do I get metabolic stress? The easiest and most often used way is through exercise. I do not mean a wimpy workout, but an endurance workout. We want these cells to be exhausting that stored glycogen. We want that lactic acid to be produced. We want cellular stress. We want you really working. That stresses the muscles but probably not your liver or kidneys that much. How about a heart attack? That will give you plenty of heart stress. Your heart is working harder with less oxygen. That will get the old autophagy going in the heart. Heart attacks do not happen that often and it would seem to be counterproductive. It's the same for a stroke. Lots of brain stress, but not that good for you.

You probably guessed it. The best way to induce generalized metabolic stress is fasting. Your body gets everyone's attention when food stops coming in. We talked about it before. Fatty acids start getting produced, ketone bodies arrive, growth hormone up, adrenalin up, cortisol up, glucagon up, and insulin down. We are preparing for metabolic war as nobody knows when we are going to eat next. This is exactly when we need autophagy. We need this body to be working as efficiently as possible. Anybody not pulling their load is ground up for energy or to make new things. Autophagy is stimulated by fasting. It gets going around 12 hours after we stop eating, the most rapid rate of increase in 12-24 hours, it peaks around 24-36 hours. These are all estimates since we cannot directly measure autophagy activity.

What stops autophagy? Why eating of course. I don't mean eating a meal, I mean eating a fourth of a meatball. Just a little protein stops autophagy. You want autophagy you have to stop eating everything. If you have been inducing autophagy a few years, it may start up faster and get to a higher peak activity. But how many of you have been fasting lately? Based on who is buying this book, no one. That is why I am going to tell you right now for the first of many times, whatever diet you are on, make sure you have at least 12 hours between your last meal and your first meal of the day. I don't care if you are on the cherry pie diet, this is a minimum. It is way too soon to try to talk you into not eating a whole day.

Think back to the last chapter. The T2DMs have been overwhelming the autophagy system with all the AGEs they are making. How many of the T2DMs do you think are fasting? After the plaques have formed in the brain, autophagy is not going to dissolve those giant structures. It works on a small scale. You must prevent the plaques; once they are there you need a different book, one that has not yet been written.

As you know, we think Alzheimer's is related to an amyloid protein. There is an enzyme that degrades amyloid before it develops plaques. This enzyme is insulin degrading enzyme (IDE). It does what it says and prefers to act on insulin. If you have high insulin, not as much left over to act on amyloid. Elevated carbs equals elevated glucose equals elevated insulin equals not as much IDE to work on amyloid. Do this for 20-30 years and you may have elevated amyloid plaques.

CHAPTER 10

KETOGENIC DIET

Tear out the previous pages of the book. This is all you need. Do any of you have actual paper pages? We have three diets to look at. (Actually, four but I was going to surprise you with the last one) These are:

Low Carb Diet

Ketogenic Diet

Fasting Diets

Believe it or not, these are not mutually exclusive.

A low carb diet is eating not as many carbs. Remember I do not know what the best diet is anymore. Throughout history, the diet has been fairly high in carbs. Something has gone wrong the last 80 or so years so that now I am going to advise a low carb diet for some. As you will see, the food has changed.

There is not a strict definition of a low carb diet, but most agree it is somewhere between 50 and 125 grams of carbohydrate a day. We do not count the fiber, so you subtract the amount of fiber from the total carbs when you a keeping your daily tallies, then eat that many carbs a day. I do not care how much fat or protein or fat you eat, just watch your carbs carefully. Now, this may or may not be a weight loss diet. This diet is primarily an insulin lowering diet. We know insulin resistance is bad news. Obesity is essentially caused by insulin resistance. Lower carbs equals lower insulin. This is the diet anyone who has had T2DM before, and by some miracle has managed to get their A1c down to normal and apparently reversed their insulin resistance, is going to be on for the rest of your life, or at least until about a month before you die. Diabetes is like alcoholism; you do not get cured. Go back to the diet you were before you got diabetes and you will get it again. Let us do some math (finally, I get to do math)

Say you are using 2100 calories a day. Remember a calorie is simply a unit of energy. We could calculate how many calories are in a barrel of oil if we wanted. For many people, 2100 calories may not be enough. It will depend on your size and amount of exercise you do. Also, somewhat on your genetics. Also, on your metabolic rate at the moment. Go back and look at the reduced calorie diet. Your metabolic rate drops.

Everyone has a set point. If you weigh 220 pounds and walk a mile, you use more calories than if you weigh 150 pounds. Overweight people get lots of exercise just in the daily activities of life. The problem is not a lack of exercise.

Anyway, carbs are 4 calories per gram, you are going to eat 150 grams then you get 600 calories a day through carbohydrates. This is a little less than a third of your daily caloric intake. If we look at something like the Mediterranean diet, and I am not saying this is the best diet, you would be getting about a third of your calories a day from each food group. So, 150 grams of carbs a day puts you in the Med diet. Of course, you need 150 grams of protein (about 5 ounces) and only 70 grams of fat (nine calories per gram).

For some reason, I have been around a lot of people on the low carb diet. I have been exposed to great meals that have been low carb. You would not know these were low carb meals. There are at least 1001 low carb cookbooks.

With the right food engineer, you would never tire of this diet. You get all the fiber you want for free; hence you can eat plenty of fruit and vegetables if you choose wisely. We are not limiting the amount of food you eat, just the amount of carbs. So, when I said you would get 150 grams of protein on the Med diet, on the low carb diet you get as much as you want. It is the same with fats. The low carb diet is not a diet in which you count calories. You do count carbs. Now you do have to use some common sense. If you eat a pound of bacon a day, you get about zero carbs, but I hope you realize this may not be wise.

The low carb diet is one you can be on for many years. Use common sense. You may or not lose weight (remember we are not counting calories), but you will most likely keep your insulin under control. It turns out that in most people, eating fat and protein tends to decrease your appetite. We may be resetting your body set weight so that it will be easier not to overeat and we can reset the historical eating by just eating when hungry and not eating when not hungry. If you have read anything in the previous chapters, you know you can shoot yourself in the foot. If you eat five 30-gram bonbons throughout the day, you are technically on the diet, but you have five insulin elevations every day. Now you are not keeping your insulin under control.

By the way, remember the 12 hours fast every day (or at least most days), and remember not to eat every hour of the day. I cannot expect most of you to go back to the twice a day historic meal plan, but at least don't go beyond three meals a day. Just maybe some of you may skip breakfast by accident. You are getting closer to fasting. If you read to the end of the chapter, I will talk about feasting.

You may ask "How come I have to be on a low carb diet now when for thousands of years nobody else had to do this?" The reason is that for thousands of years everyone did not have insulin resistance. Something has screwed us up and now we cannot go back to the traditional higher carb diet. We can talk about it later as to what has happened, but the fact remains the modern western diet, is different from the historical diet.

It also may be that although there was plenty of food, people still did not eat as many calories as they do today. If you eat carbs, the liver will begin turning excess glucose into triglycerides. If there isn't that much excess glucose, the triglycerides won't go up as much. This may also be a factor in reducing obesity. As we talked about earlier, there is the factor of processed food. For various reasons, this does increase the insulin problem.

The ketogenic diet is one in which you are spilling ketone bodies in your urine. There is only one main ketone body which is beta-hydroxybutyric acid (BHB). This is produced about the same time glucose is being produced by the liver after fatty acid production by the fat cells has begun. Ketones can be used as a source of energy by almost everyone in the body including the brain. The brain also uses ketones to make long chain fatty acids. Ketones sound great and they are rather good. Not quite as energy rich as fatty acids but useful.   By the way, one reason the brain does not use fatty acids is that they are too fat to get past the blood-brain barrier. Ketones are much smaller.

So how do you know if you are spilling ketones in the urine? You go down and buy the keto urine sticks. Anything greater than negative means you are spilling ketones. What does that mean? You may have a very low level of ketones in the urine all the time. Remember most metabolic processes never go all the way down to zero. We have arbitrarily drawn a line and said that 4.0 is the level that you are in ketosis. This turns out to be the first level above zero on most keto urine sticks. Probably 99% of the sticks are purchased by people who want to check to see if they are in ketogenesis.

By now you have already figured out what it is and how to get there. Insulin and glucagon are the determinants of which fatty acid process the fat cells are being driven. By now you also know carbohydrate is the driver of insulin secretion. So logically you need to decrease the number of carbs in your diet. This sounds easy enough.

On the low carb diet, you ate no more than about 150 grams of carbs a day. Occasionally you would eat more and sometimes less but you would try to not go much higher. If we were going to measure something to see if this was working, it would be the A1c if you started on this diet to help or prevent T2DM, or your weight if you kind of wanted to lose weight. The low carb diet will often provide some weight loss, especially if you currently are on a high carb diet. It is quite possible you will eventually begin to lower your set point and your body will naturally lower your weight just by restoring the normal weight control mechanisms.

For many years you did not have to pay any particular attention to your weight and maintained a constant level. Over time you were able to mess that up, primarily through an elevated carbohydrate diet. Hopefully, that can be restored. A low carb diet is more in the category of a maintenance diet, that you and your family can be on for years. A ketogenic diet is a weight loss diet. You cannot be on this for years.

To get in ketogenesis you will have to lower your carbs down to about 25 grams. This is an estimate since people are different. Not only that but this level changes as time goes on. Lowering your carbs induces metabolic changes in your body such that it may be easier to get into ketogenesis. The number of carbs necessary to maintain ketogenesis may vary as time goes on. We do not care about the exact number, as long as the stick turns positive. You do not have to count carbs, you just know you need a low level, and if the stick is not positive, you need to lower the level.

Ketogenesis does not happen instantly. Even if you ate zero carbohydrates, it takes a few days, maybe 2-4. You must eventually get there. If not, you are doing something wrong. Everyone can put an app on their cell phones to find out carbs in what they eat. Most food has it written right on the package. Take the total carbs and subtract the fiber. You get the number of carbs. Keep going lower until you get a positive stick. After a while, you will be able to figure out the carb intake without thinking too much about it. Let us go through some details.

At this point I need in interject something. The point of the low carb diet is not to get into ketogenesis, although if you did it would be no big deal. Often people on the low carb diet will go far lower than 150 grams.

Speaking of 150 grams, some will have to go lower than this. We are on the low carb diet to control insulin. We are aiming to get our HgbA1c into the lower range. If you cannot do that with 150 grams, you will have to go lower. Once you get to prediabetes, we must get your A1c down. Afterall, you had to have an elevated A1c to get that diagnosis. Keep lowering the carbs still your A1c is normal.

If it never gets normal, stay on the low carb diet, but now you may need some medication. It's possible you may be at the point that you are actually getting low on insulin. Now we have a different problem.

CHAPTER 11

<u>DIET DETAILS</u>

The advantage of the ketogenic diet is that you get to eat. You just do not get to eat carbs. Everyone has heard of people putting butter on steak or eating pork rinds or eating bacon and eggs for breakfast and lunch every day; these stories are true. Ketogenesis means your fat cells are putting out fatty acids. Your fat cells are not turning sugar into fat. This will be happening as long as your stick is positive.

Now if you eat a lot of triglycerides (fat) and absorb a lot of fatty acids, your body is happy to use these also. This may slow down the rate your fat cells put out fatty acids, but if your carb level is low, it is not turning sugar into fat. OK, some of you caught me. Even if you are not eating carbs, your dutiful liver is still making sugar out of protein. Your blood sugar level may drop a little, but it will not go to zero. Your brain does not mind using ketone bodies, but not for 100% of its energy. You will always have some blood sugar from your liver, even if you are fasting for months. There may be a little sugar going to fat but at a much lower rate than before you bought this book. In fact, at such a low rate we are going to forget about it.

The main advantage of this diet over say the reduced calorie diet is that you may eat protein and fat; almost as much as you want. You still can't go crazy as people are wont to do, but if you use your common sense, you can eat butter and steak and lobster. This may be a fat loss diet but will not be a cheap diet. Your hunger will not be a driver for eating. You will eat when you get hungry. Now there are other advantages to not eating all the time other than just insulin control which we can talk about later. What about cholesterol? Well, it may go up a little. It may not, depending upon how poor your previous diet was. The ketogenic diet is a fat losing diet. I have told you several times this is not a maintenance diet. You would be crazy (not medical advice) if you continue this diet forever.

If we say most bought the book to lose about 30 pounds, this will take about 3-6 months, everybody is different. We are going to determine that the risk-benefit ratio is going to be in favor of our lowering weight versus the possible risks of a high protein/fat diet. This is true for most people, but not everyone. There may or may not be an increased risk of kidney stones or gout, especially if you are already afflicted by this. Yes, your lipoprotein profile may look a little worse, but it may not. We are losing weight. If we had not screwed up by gaining weight, all this would not have been necessary. Now we are trying to fix it and we have calculated the fix is better than the disease. I am not a health care provider. If you are not a normal person health-wise going into this, maybe you should see some type of health care provider. Then it's their fault and not mine if something goes amiss.

We are on our way to fat loss heaven. What could possibly go wrong? It ends up when you switch from glucose to fatty acids, sometimes you may not feel great for a couple of days. You remember what happens when you stop eating. The glycogen gets used up, the fatty acids get started, the ketones get started and the liver sugar making gets going. This process is in flux. Sometimes you may feel a little hypoglycemic. Sometimes you may feel a little low energy. Sometimes you don't feel quite right. My approach is that is just too bad. At least you are not hungry. Remember there is a reason we are doing this whole thing. Somehow you managed to gain a lot of fat. Maybe you may have to feel not bad, just not normal for a couple of days. This will pass. You have lots of energy stored in your body. Your liver will make glucose for you. The fatty acids will get turned into ketone bodies for you. Suck it up.

One problem is psychological. You are addicted to sucrose and high fructose corn syrup, and we are going cold turkey. You will have some withdrawal symptoms. Again, too bad. We are going all Calvinistic on you. Eat some pork rinds.

We do end up in ketosis. Our ketosis flu does go away. We are now ordering the low carb lunches, counting all our carbs, eating about three times a day, fasting for 12 hours between the last and first meals, and everyone we talk to knows what you are saying when you say, "I am going low carb". So far so good. Oft times people get a slight euphoria. It would not be surprising if you wanted to start exercising or join the YMCA. I encourage this activity, not because I believe exercise greatly helps weight loss, although I believe it does encourage certain metabolic processes, but because half the people there are in the same boat as you.

There is something to group support and peer pressure. There is an advantage to being around people who will encourage you and give good advice. Don't be shy. Everyone supports someone who has taken the step to health and self-improvement. Most were there once and understand changing your life is not easy, but possible. Commit to an exercise class. I believe the psychological advantage is much more than the physical. Stay in ketosis and you will lose fat. It will just be more fun if you are around similar people.

One of the unexpected problems of a very low carb diet is that it gets boring. I am sure in the past people got tired of eating buffalo every day in the summer or a potato every day in the winter, but it was better than being hungry. We have a slight advantage now. The capitalistic system has provided us with thousands of low carb recipes. Many are excellent dishes that no one would know was low carb. Many are recipes you may have never made before. With a little effort, the food engineer can give you enough variety that boredom should not be a problem.

This is opposed to cravings. Normally I treat men and women the same, often with little sympathy and generally with tough love. This is one area that may be physiologic. Both men and women get cravings. Women for food, men for something else. The cravings in pregnancy are a real physiologic event that, if we were smart enough, could see actual brain changes. The relationship between food desire and the brain is some combination of hormones, gut bacteria, previous exposure, and physiology.

I will sympathize with the desire for carbs, but you cannot succumb. Exercise may help this. The stimulation of the other taste buds may relieve some of the pressure. In pregnancy, the craving may be dill pickles as much as ice cream. You have five taste buds; try to stimulate others to control the sweet desire. Salty pork rinds, steak with lots of mushrooms, chili peppers: you are not alone here, and recipe books can be of great benefit.

You can see this diet is somewhat bereft of vegetables and fiber. Spend what few carbs you have wisely. Fiber does not count. You will also be a little light on fruit. For most of history, man ate fruit only a few months a year. You should be able to last six months. Eating fruit every day of the year is not normal. You will be fine. This is a fat -loss diet, not a lifelong maintenance diet.

I hesitate to tell you this, but I hope you will use common sense with this information. It is probably not good for you to be in ketosis all the time. Being in ketosis results in a low insulin level. That is what we are trying to accomplish. Ketosis all the time is not a normal metabolic state.

We are putting up with it for a while because we calculated the risk was worth the benefit. Insulin affects other hormones as well as carbohydrates. Your body is very complex with hormones, organs, and brain elaborately connected. It ends up that to keep all the hormones happy, we may have to go out of ketosis every few weeks. By that I mean every three to four weeks you will eat an elevated carb meal. I don't mean you go crazy, but maybe you go to a Mexican restaurant and order off the regular menu. This will take you out of ketosis.

The next day can go back to the diet. In a day or two, you will be back on the wagon with the keto sticks. This recommendation is not gospel. It is difficult for me to find a lot of medical research support. I'm pretty sure it won't hurt you and it will only prolong your weight loss diet for a short time. Your hormones have a rhythm.

Now relax and have an open mind. Do not be afraid. We are going to start the next chapter and it will be scary for some people.

CHAPTER 12

FASTING

Fasting is no caloric intake. For practical purposes, if it is less than one, we are going to call it zero. Although there is fasting in which you have no intake at all, as in not even water, we are not doing that. I do not even recommend that unless there happens to be some religious element involved. This is not medical advice, just common sense.

Starvation is no caloric intake in the absence of fat reserves. We are not doing that. I do not recommend that at all either. Of course, most people in a starvation state are not there by choice.

Like the other diets we have considered, both fasting and starvation are completely different metabolic states with different processes going on. We have already discussed what happens when we stop eating. We have already agreed (maybe) to not eat between the last meal and the first meal as a method of insulin control and to induce autophagy. All types of other things happen when you stop eating.

First, let us agree that fasting is not some type of fad. Fasting has existed throughout recorded history. It has often been used as a method to enhance the body's natural healing processes. It appears the human body is designed to incorporate fasting as a normal homeostatic process. Hippocrates the father of medicine recommended fasting as did many of the great minds of history. In the 1920s there were fasting clinics in the United States and Europe treating hundreds of thousands of patients with various medical problems. It is not weird. At the same time, we must use a little common sense. I do not think we would treat a broken leg with fasting; nevertheless, hold off on any judgment till you hear me out.

We already know that in fasting the insulin goes down; the glucagon goes up, cortisol, growth hormone, and adrenalin all up. After a little while, fatty acids up, glucose manufacturing up, and ketones up. After 24 hours the metabolism is up. Another 24 hours and it is up again. Remember that autophagy. Just a little bit of protein stops it. Enough carbs will also stop it by increasing insulin. Around 36 hours we reach our maximum autophagy. It now continues plugging along as long as we are fasting. Remember autophagy is converting some of the cellular trash into energy. It is doing what it takes to keep the cell alive and at peak efficiency. Now we have reached a stable metabolic state and we can keep going as long as the fat holds out.

For the most part, when people think of fasting, they think of therapeutic fasting, which is fasting to lose a specific amount of weight, not fasting as part of your normal diet. This is the most rapid way to lose weight. It ends up being up to about 0.7 pounds a day. You may think this is crazy to do that, but not really. Say you have to fit into your wedding dress in three weeks and you need to get rid of ten pounds of fat. What keeps you from just not eating? We already discussed that for most people it would not be unhealthy. In fact, after looking through the benefits of fasting, maybe you would end up healthier. The only thing that holds anyone back from not doing this more often is motivation and fear. A bride with a wedding dress to wear in three weeks has tons of motivation and no fear of a little fasting.

I will divide fasting up into therapeutic (designed for weight loss, and homeostatic (designed to be part of your normal diet for health promotion). There is also religious fasting that I will not cover here.

Therapeutic fasting is just not eating for a period of time. As long as you have plenty of fat stores, you will not get into a starvation state. After a few days, your metabolism stabilizes. As you recall, your body is preparing you to get food. An increase in growth hormone spares your skeletal muscle because you are going to need that to get food. Your metabolism rises because you are going to need that energy to get food. Also, fasting stimulates ghrelin. This is a hormone that is connected to the brain. It probably increases concentration, memory, and attention. These are all factors that will be important to you so that you can find more food.

We need a little more info on leptin and ghrelin. As we know, leptin is elevated when we are full. You can get leptin resistance just like insulin resistance and T2DMs may have a chronic elevation of leptin without the effect of being full. Likewise, when ghrelin is elevated you are hungry. Like many hormones in the human body, there is a rhythm to the secretion of these hormones. The actual peaks may vary up and down, but the hormones are somewhat pulsatile. It turns out ghrelin also has a circadian rhythm. It rises about three times a day, lasts about two hours, and then falls. As fasting goes on the pulsatile secretion continues but the peak level falls.

This explains the common experience of decreasing hunger as fasting goes on. Hunger does not continue to increase but falls to a low level. It appears we are designed to experience hunger periodically. Just like it appears we need to fast every now and then to promote autophagy. It also appears humans have an innate fear of fasting. Maybe it would be more correct to say an instinct to avoid starvation.

You often hear people say they are starving. I doubt they are really in a starvation metabolic state, but that is an expression of the fear of starving. It is difficult for people to imagine fasting for three days. They say they just cannot do it, that they would get too hungry or that they would be unable to walk for lack of energy. None of these are true. Fasting does require one to overcome a natural fear, yet it can be done. At least let's agree it is not a crazy thing to do and work up to it.

Fasting has become popular to the point that now we have names for a few of them:

There is not a name for our 12 hours fast between the last meal and first meal. This is a normal part of life and we should be doing this most of the time.

16:8 fast: You eat 8 hours a day and fast 16 hours. This is essentially your normal diet and skipping breakfast. You end up eating 2-3 meals a day. This extends your autophagy a little longer and induces your fatty acid creation a little. Induction of these adaptive metabolic processes takes quite a while. The longer you do this, the faster the fatty acids get going. It also limits your eating to eight hours a day.

20:4 fast: You eat four hours a day. This is also called the warrior diet as I imagine during times of conflict people ended up doing this anyway. The eating was usually in the evening. Maybe you should try this on Thanksgiving.

OMAD fast: Eating one meal a day. You eat supper and then don't eat till supper the next day. I'm sure many have done this by necessity at times. What you may have noticed is that you may get hungry during the day, but it comes and goes. Perhaps this is related to the cyclical secretion of ghrelin for a couple of hours. If you just wait for a little while, the hunger goes away. Good confidence builder

5:2 fast: for two non-consecutive days a week you don't eat. This is a combination weight loss and health promotion diet. Make sure you eat normally (as in eating till you are full and do not fill your meals with junk food) on the days you are eating. Do not try to combine this with a reduced calorie diet by trying to eat less on your eat days. You will just get all the worst characteristics of the most failed diet. Eat normally on eat days.

Long fasts: By that, I mean longer than three weeks. Remember we do not want a starvation metabolic state. If you lose 0.7 pounds a day for 21 days, that's about 12-

15 pounds. Make sure you have 12-15 pounds of fat. If you want long fasts, that are greater than 21 days, maybe you need medical advice. I am not giving you any. See next chapter.

People are afraid to fast. You can see how we can build up to it. You are already fasting at least 12 hours a day. It's easy to skip breakfast. You get a little hunger at lunch but before you know it, you are on the OMAD fast

The 5:2 fast has become popular. You just eat your normal diet except two days a week when you do not eat. There is no extra counting. You have 36 hours of fasting which will put many into ketosis and maximize your autophagy. You can do this fast one or two days a week with any other diet. It may help if you are stuck on a certain weight and need a jump start. You can do this with your maintenance diet. If you have a history of T2DM and now are on your lifetime lower carbohydrate diet, you can always throw this in.

Say you have been doing this for a year. Would you be afraid not to eat for a few days? Not that you should do this, but certainly you won't worry about it too much if you were in a situation where you couldn't eat for a couple of days.

Next is a real-life story that gives us insight into the human body. I am not advising anyone to do this, but this is what happens if you do.

CHAPTER 13

ANGUS FAST

Angus Barbieri entered a Scottish hospital in June 1965 for a 3-week fast. At that time, he weighed 465 pounds. Fasting as a treatment for various diseases has been used for thousands of years. Angus wanted to lose weight and fasting was considered to be an appropriate treatment. After three weeks he was doing well and wanted to continue the fast. His doctors agreed and he returned to the hospital regularly over the next year. In all, he fasted for 382 days and stopped when he reached his goal weight of 180 pounds. One of the significant aspects of this fast is the medical documentation and in fact, a case study was published in 1973.

Stewart, WK., Fleming, LW (1973) Features of a successful therapeutic fast of 382 days duration: Postgraduate *Medical Journal, 49(569), 203-209*

He lost an average of 0.7 pounds a day. During the fast, he was given vitamin supplements, and for a few months added potassium supplements. For most of the fast, his blood glucose was about 30 mg/dl. There is much to take away from this fast but for our purposes a few important facts. He did not get continually hungrier throughout the fast; in fact, he reported what many others have stated that his hunger went away. His weight loss of about 0.7 pounds a day is consistent with other observations and would be considered the upper level of weight loss in fasting.

He had no significant medical issues and, for a short fast of a few weeks, it seems there should be no problems for most people. He was remarkably tolerant of the low glucose levels. His glucose levels were derived solely from what he was making out of protein. Remember he started with a lot of protein as well as fat. It took a lot more tissue to support a 465-pound man versus a 180-pound man. This protein was metabolized to not only make glucose but also to provide all the minerals and electrolytes he needed.

The pictures at the end do not show a man with skin sagging all over the place, but rather a normal-looking person. One can assume the excess skin was also metabolized and used as well as the excess muscle, bone, and constituents of the other organs. A man weighing 465 pounds needs larger organs everywhere than a 180-pound man and his body was able to adjust the amount of bone, muscle heart, liver, kidney, and other organs to the appropriate size for his weight.

Now, this occurred with fasting. I cannot say the same thing would occur if you were eating, such as someone who had bariatric surgery. They are not fasting but are taking in protein and carbs. There does seem to be some skin sagging on these people.

They did monitor him for a little while after he started eating. His blood sugar went back to normal.

Let me emphasize this was a fast, which is a different metabolic state than ketogenesis, which is a different metabolic state than starvation, which is a different metabolic state than a reduced calorie diet, which is a different metabolic state than a maintenance diet, which is a different metabolic state than a low carbohydrate diet.

I have found this concept to be difficult to adjust to for most people. Also fasting is a normal mechanism, not this much fasting, but certainly for a day or so. It is necessary to promote autophagy and normal homeostasis. A weight loss fast is a therapeutic fast, not a normal part of your diet. Similarly, the ketogenic diet is a weight loss diet, not a maintenance diet. Just like it would not be healthy to be on a fast all of your life, it is not healthy to be in ketogenesis all your life. It is a therapeutic weight loss diet and needs to come to an end eventually.

The nerds among us can check out the case study. I picked up something when I read it again today. His cholesterol started at 230; it didn't change any. So much for the low-fat diet.

CHAPTER 14

MAINTENANCE DIET

Let us say you have succeeded. You have lost fat. As we look back, we understand what happened. We stayed in ketogenesis most of the time and we knew we did because we were checking the stick. The sticks do not lie. If we weren't in keto, it was because we were eating too many carbs. We know what carbs are by now and everyone could tell me how many carbs are in a roll. We were eating fat and protein. Eventually, we even got bored of eating fat and protein. But at least we did not have a continuing issue with hunger like the reduced calorie diet and we should have had enough energy. Sure, we had occasional plateaus of no weight loss, but we stuck to it and eventually achieved the goal. Everybody did not make it.

This diet does not usually fail if you remain in ketosis. You can subvert this by eating a whole lot of fat and protein even while remaining in ketosis. As we stated, this is not usually a problem as your appetite diminishes somewhat, but some do manage to do this.

The most common cause of failure is mental. We need to recognize there is a craving for sweets in humans. This is a sort of addiction that some cannot overcome, just like opioids or nicotine. It varies with personalities and circumstances, but just like some people will continue smoking despite a heart attack, some cannot overcome the desire for sweets. It's not hunger, but rather some other need for which carbs supply the cure. We can wait for a better mental state or resolution of some anxiety or depressive disorder and try again. This can be one of the side effects of excessive artificial sweeteners.

For many, this has worked. You have lost fat. Often this is associated with increased physical activities. The diet made you lose weight, not physical activity. Do not fall into the trap that the reason I am not losing weight or am gaining weight is that I am not exercising enough. Exercise will increase your ability to work, but it will not usually make you lose fat unless it is accompanied by a good maintenance diet.

Now what? Somehow, we got into this situation of being 20-pound overweight and now we have finally lost the fat. I bet that if you go back to the same diet you had, you will return to the 20-pound overweight status. More importantly, if you lost the fat because you were concerned about your increased risk of developing diabetes, I can guarantee you will circle back around to your previous state if you return to your previous diet. You cannot be on ketosis forever so let me give you some options here. Sometimes you have an alcoholic who can go back to drinking a little, but you have to be careful.

The maintenance diet is one we can live with for 30 years. Sure, we have occasions for feasting and periods that fasting may be wise, but for almost all the time we can stick to it. We need one suitable for everyone who is at the table, be they 7 or 70. We would like to be able to eat until we are not hungry. This was the way you used to do it until your weight set point went amiss. For many years you ate till you were finished eating and your weight barely varied. If you exerted more energy, or if you were sedentary, your body adjusted your appetite to the right intake to maintain homeostasis. If you are a growing teenager, you will eat more without anyone telling you to. If you are a sedentary older person, you will eat less than when you were doing physical labor. You did not have to calculate anything, your body naturally adjusted.

It would be nice if we could just go back to the common diet over the last several thousand years where people ate what they had. This varied according to the seasons and area, but most had plenty of food. Like now they sometimes became bored with their diet, but there was no obesity epidemic. Something has happened in the last 100 years so that now we can't do that anymore. Diabetes, obesity, and autoimmune disease are all increasing. Just like the past, there is no lack of food, but somehow the food is affecting us differently and the environment has changed. Something is amiss.

In times past, the carb load was about 50-60% of the calories, especially when it was necessary to rely on stored food. For some reason we cannot do that now, my thoughts next chapter on why. I believe we do need a different ratio, something like the Mediterranean diet we discussed earlier. We need to lower the total carbs to somewhere between 25-35% of the diet. Why? The modern carbs are different. That leaves us with protein and fat. Let's divided these up about 50/50. Now we have a little less than a third of our diet carbs, about a third protein, and about a little more than a third fat. The next chapter will be how to divide these up.

Now the 12 hours fast every day. I need to insist on that. I believe for homeostasis, insulin control, hormonal regulation, circadian rhythms, sleep, and all kinds of other reasons, your body was designed with this in mind. In fact, for thousands of years, this was the norm. Go back to twelve hours between the last meal and the first. No snacking. No calories. You must trust me on this one. This may be one of the most important aspects of the maintenance diet.

Eating twice a day was the norm for most of history. I think this is not a bad idea, but in today's environment, modern life does not lend itself to this practice. If I can get you to agree to only eat three times a day, it will be a great success. That means no donut at 10:00 am, no power bar at 3:00 pm, no whey protein shakes after a workout. Exercise, eating, and bodybuilding is another book. It will not make me popular. With the advent of artificial lighting, I am resigned to people eating after sundown which makes three meals a day to be the natural rhythm of eating. For me, I don't mind skipping lunch.

We have an outline. The food engineer is now the central element in health. This person has to choose the food. It is a difficult process now with many pitfalls. They must prepare the food which dictates as to when people are going to eat and how much there is to eat. I always advise enough food. The worst practical diet is the reduced calorie diet. At the same time, you do not what to have a bunch of food left over (unless you are roasting a whole pig) that may encourage midnight eating.

It is a complicated process to know how much to prepare and to use food wisely. If you are doing this correctly, there probably will be a little left over after every meal. The engineer must balance the carbs/fats/proteins, must prepare food correctly and appealingly, must know what most people will eat, must serve a wide age range, must ensure food safety in preparation and storage, and must do this on a budget.

They must do this 2-3 times a day almost every day of the year. The alternative is to eat out somewhere or order food from somewhere. These people you order food from are preparing the food so that you order it again. This usually is not to your advantage. If you buy previously prepared and packaged food, you are getting preservatives and additives. I do not trust these are all safe. Many others do not either. Ideally, food is fresh and not preserved, but we have been eating preserved food for thousands of years. Sometimes we just ate potatoes every day because that was all there was.

As you can see, the food engineer is a full-time job. It requires years of practice, continuing education, and experience to do a good job. Maybe we should get in the habit of letting the food engineer off one day a week. Maybe we should stop making the food engineer work a second job.

Maintenance Diet: We have 12 hours fast, 2-3 meals a day, about a third of our calories from each food group, fresh food, try to be careful when we eat out and do not do this often. Everyone at the adult table eats the same. Young kids have different requirements. Use your common sense. Eat more vegetables than grains. Try to eliminate HFCS and decrease sucrose to a minimum. That will allow you to eat fruit without having to worry about a fructose burden.

This is it. Now you can throw away (?) the book. Or maybe you want a few more details and some juicy speculation. If so, read on a couple more chapters although I anticipate most will stop here. I hope the food engineers continue.

I have addressed the issue of a maintenance diet in another book , *Maintenance Diet for the Modern Man*, which was written specifically for the food engineer.

CHAPTER 15

KILLER SUGAR

Why are we getting fat in the last 100 years as opposed to the last 5000? I agree that throughout history there have been a few fat people, but these were not common. In fact, 2500 years ago it was noted that there were two types of diabetes: one associated with youth and one with obesity. These cases were quite rare. The pathogenesis of diabetes was not uncovered until about 1920. The worldwide incidence of T2DM has increased from 25 million to 300 million since 1985. The incidence of diabetes in the USA in 1958 was 1%. The incidence now is 10%. The incidence of prediabetes, which we can call obesity, is 40%.

I give up trying to figure out the number of overweight people or even what overweight means. In about 60 years, we have gone from 10 % diabetes to 40% diabetes and prediabetes. The graph is still going up, not only in the USA but around the world.

I do not even want to calculate how much this is costing the health care system which for the most part, I am paying for. I believe this is getting into black plaque territory and we can officially call this an epidemic.

Something or maybe several things happened in the last 100 years to make us get fat. Remember it was not just more available food. Other than sporadic episodes of government-induced famine (Depression, world wars), food has been readily available over the last few thousand years. Maybe it's the type of food. I am biased so I am saying it is. He is my reasoning.

Average sucrose consumption USA per day

1700   1 teaspoon

1800   4 teaspoons

1900   28 teaspoons

2009   50% of USA ate 52 teaspoons a day

About 16 calories per teaspoon so about 600 calories a day in sucrose.

What is so special about sucrose as opposed to a potato which is full of starch containing a bunch of glucose? Mainly it is that sucrose is composed of half glucose and half fructose. It is also absorbed rapidly. It doesn't take much to split the sucrose into glucose and fructose. This is done more rapidly if the sucrose is already hydrated, which means it is already dissolved in water. The glucose has a great absorption system as your body is greedy for energy and does not want any sugar to escape in the stool. The glucose goes straight to the liver which rapidly dumps it into the blood.

Same deal with fructose. Still rapid but not as much as glucose. The liver does not dump this directly into the blood but changes it first. It manages to handle most of it, but the larger the load and more rapidly it is absorbed, the less time the liver has to metabolize fructose, and the more that is released into the bloodstream. The glucose skips this metabolizing step.

Historically most of our carbs were not already dissolved sucrose. Fructose was bound up with fiber and had to be released to get absorbed. Glucose was bound up in large starch molecules and had to be converted to maltose and then to glucose. These had to be dissolved also. For almost all our history the liver was given plenty of time to metabolize the fructose and more slowly distribute the glucose. As a result, the glucose level did not rise as rapidly or go as high. Even though the total amount of glucose ingestion was about the same, it was in the form of starch and not dissolved glucose. Although the exposure was the same, the rise in insulin was not.

Honey is a good example. It contains free fructose and free glucose. It still must be hydrated to be absorbed. Also, it works out that food can be too sweet. Fructose is sweeter than glucose; hence it is not that easy to eat a tablespoon of honey. Glucose is sweeter than maltose; hence you can eat a tablespoon of starch much easier than a tablespoon of sugar.

So, although the carb intake is the same as 5000 years ago, the rate of glucose rising in the blood is faster, and the initial surge of insulin is higher. It probably also causes the total amount under the curve (the accumulated total secretion) of insulin to be slightly higher. Not much, but after a couple hundred thousand times (40 years), it may be enough to induce insulin resistance.

What is high fructose corn syrup (HFCS)? Start with corn, take off the kernels, crush these up. Now you make a vat full of corn starch. Remember this is just a bunch of starch, which is a long chain of glucose. Now you mix in an enzyme which breaks the bonds, so you have a bunch of maltose molecules, now you add an enzyme that breaks it down to a bunch of glucose molecules. Add water and now you have Karo Corn Syrup, which is basically glucose honey. (But not as sweet) Now you can take a vat of Karo Corn Syrup, add some enzymes, and you get a vat of fructose instead of a vat of glucose. Why would anyone want to do that? Well around 1984 the soda pop companies decided to begin using HFCS as the sweetener instead of sucrose. To get the same sweetness for pop you mix 55 parts of fructose with 45 parts of glucose. In food products, it is a 42/58 ratio.

Why would the pop companies do that? To protect the US sugar industry, tariffs were placed on sugar imports. Now it was cheaper to use HFCS. First the low-fat diet, now HFCS. I wonder why people don't trust the government. I wonder if the best scientists work for the government or private industry.

Now we are eating pure fructose and glucose, already in a liquid form. Essentially, we are mainlining heroin. The liver gets bombed by a load of this stuff. It goes ahead and dumps the glucose into the blood, perhaps at a slightly higher rate than if it was from sucrose, and the peak may be marginally higher. The fructose overwhelms the livers capacity to metabolize it. The body does not have to separate the fructose from the fiber; it gets absorbed rapidly to the liver. This process allows more fructose to float around in your blood than was historically present. It also gives us a larger total burden of fructose than the historical diet.

When it just came from fruits, fructose was seasonal, and the total yearly burden was less. Now fructose consumption is about five times higher than 100 years ago. I have already advised you of the much greater proclivity of fructose to form AGEs and how we consider these to be the primary drivers of aging and dementia, HFCS has also been associated with increased T2DM, cancer growth, fatty liver, elevated cholesterol, hypertension, and leaky gut (next chapter).

The incidence of all of these side effects is rising. I cannot say that HFCS is the cause of this rise, but I can say that HFCS has not been a part of the human diet for 99% of recorded history. And I can say that US consumption per year per capita went from zero in 1975 to 40 pounds a year now. At this point, it may be that the primary source of triglycerides in the body is not from the fat we eat, but rather from the fructose that has been converted o triglyceride in the liver. The liver now needs to make a bunch of lipoproteins to transport this triglyceride to the rest of the body. See addendum.

Food engineer, please cut back on HFCS and sucrose Also remember that for most of man's history, they did not eat fruit every day.

CHAPTER 16

<u>KILLER GRAINS</u>

I can see how sugar may not be good for you but not bread! Come on. People have been eating bread for 5000 years. How can that be bad for you?

I agree. How can grains, which have been used for calories and as a way to preserve food, possibly be contributing to the current epidemic of obesity? Maybe something has changed.

Most people generally recognize about six ancient grains that have been motioned or used thousands of years ago. This grain has changed throughout history through crossbreeding. I have noted that each generation believes they are much smarter than the previous one. Today we know how to use a cell phone. Does anyone know how to fix them? Do you know how they work? Do you know how to make a circuit board or even a single transistor? Do you have any idea where to find a particular rock that if crushed (do you know how to crush it) and processed (how do you do that) and finally extract an ore that needs to be combined with several others to make a teeny part of an electrical connection that connects with a thousand others? Somehow the past generation figured out how to do that.

In the same manner, crossbreeding of crops and animals have been around for 5000 years. Do you think that just because they did not know what DNA was that they couldn't figure out that if I breed this small plant enough times, eventually all the plants will be small? This was initially used to increase production or make the plants resistant to certain diseases or to be able to grow in certain environments.

This took a long time, but as civilizations developed, more variety of plants were available, and the crossbreeding continued to the point that the different grains today are unlike the same species 5000 years ago. The prime example is the dwarfing of wheat by Norman Borlaug. In 1944 he went to Mexico to breed wheat. Fertilizers applied to wheat made them grow, but taller wheat and more grain caused them to fall to the ground and rot. Through several years of crossbreeding, he developed dwarf wheat (he also developed other traits in this dwarf wheat) that enabled a great increase in productivity, partially by being able to fertilize the wheat without making it fall over from being too tall. In 1960 Mexico became a net exporter of wheat for the first time. This same process was repeated in India and Southeast Asia. Now 95% of the wheat we eat is a dwarf variety. No such thing existed 2000 years ago.

The nutritional components are different, the amount of gluten different, protein different. It may have the same basic gene makeup, but it is different wheat designed for productivity, not the natural variety initially on the earth. Now more land is devoted to growing wheat than all other crops combined. This is an example of capitalism at its finest, just like HFCS. We have plenty of food, but it is not the same. If we are looking for something that has changed the food supply in the last 75 years, this could be it.

One more thing. Not only is the wheat different, but the processing is different. For thousands of years, stone milling was used. Wheat kernels have a hard covering. Flour is the soft part (endosperm) in the middle. To get to the flour we have to crush the bran and separate it from the endosperm. This is stone milling. A big stone in a circle crushed whatever it rolled over. The bran was separated, and the rest used. Some stones crushed it finer and this made it easier to use. Over the thousands of years, we have gotten better at crushing the wheat, till now it is very fine. I mean getting to the size of a blood cell fine.

Most are larger than that, but fine flour is about 8 times larger than a red blood cell. This is about 50 to 100 times smaller than the historical average.

What is the effect of this? Well, we increase the surface area of the flour 1000-10,000 times. Remember when that starch took longer to break down into its glucose subunits and thus spread out the time it took to absorb the glucose from carbs, well now we have done the same thing to wheat as we do with HFCS in that the glucose is absorbed faster and the peak slightly higher: all leading to more total insulin and, you guessed it, more insulin resistance. Of course, you realize everything I have said could be called speculation, and it is: but most ideas start as speculation. Time will tell.

European bread is baked daily with no additives. Supermarket bread has additives and preservatives. I am not sure this is good for you or just the supermarket.

The preservatives are present to prevent bacterial and mold growth.   Do you think that may be affecting your gut biome?

I go into detail in another book, *Bread in the Modern Diet.*

CHAPTER 17

OUR GUT FRIENDS

The human microbiome is the collection of bacteria, viruses, parasites, and other organisms that live with and on us. There are lots of these. Each area of your body has a different collection. Your ear canal, scalp, eyebrows, mouth, armpit, gut, belly button, vagina, and penis, foot: all have their different collection which is also different among all individuals. We are interested in the gut.

The gut microbiome is also different for each individual and depends on where you live. Each area of the country has a different collection that may be similar, although not identical to your neighbor. Most of the bacteria do not change over time unless something happens. That something that happens could be the ingestion of some medicine or chemical that could affect bacteria. Different food can slightly affect the biome.

The biome is important as this is part of the barrier in the gut between the bad world outside and the nice world inside of you. Your gut is the immunological battleground for activating your immune system. Your gut lining must decide all the time whether to allow substances to enter your body or not. Upon entering our body, any proteins are identified as friend or foe and acted upon appropriately. Remember your gut is digesting everything you eat and breaking fats and proteins down into their individual parts. Sometimes the proteins are not broken down completely and a piece enters the body to be confronted by the immune system.

Sometimes these get into the blood and travel around. The gut wall usually has a tight junction between cells and is selective about what it lets in, but nothing works perfectly so the immune system is always on standby. The bacteria in the gut help us with digestion, eliminating harmful bacteria, and preventing the growth of other harmful bacteria.

In return, we provide them with various nutrients. Although in the previous chapters I have spoken about the absorption of various nutrients, it is not a perfect process and carbs, fats, and protein do sometimes avoid being absorbed and the bacteria have access to these sometimes partially digested nutrients.

So why am I telling all this useful but seemingly irrelevant information? Well, this may be part of the problem associated with our diet in the last 60 years. It appears that different bacteria are associated with different diseases. People with T2DM have an abnormal gut biome. If we transfer some of their gut bacteria into mice, the mice end up with T2DM; it's the same with some other diseases. Then we have immune problems like gluten sensitivity or other autoimmune diseases.

We know diseases like obesity and diabetes, have also been increasing in the last 60 years. For immune disease, the increase is in certain parts of the world, just like the microbiome is different in certain parts of the world.

Some of us get a "leaky gut" in which more proteins than normal slip through the gut cell walls and may stimulate the immune system. Some of these proteins or parts of protein may resemble other parts of your body enough that you end up getting the immune system riled up against yourself. By the way, I didn't invent this idea, but it is intriguing. If I connect the dots, the leaky gut may be associated with an abnormal gut biome.

An abnormal gut biome is associated with antibiotics and other medications. But it may also be associated with small amounts of other chemicals we have been picking up over the last 60 years like pesticides on food, insecticides, herbicides, Roundup, fertilizers, trace chemicals in the environment: All elements that have become more common in our industrial crop raising environment and all have increased over the last 60 years. I am including food additives and preservatives. So why am I telling you this?

Food engineer, please notice. I believe that overall, organically raised food has less of this than non-organic. For some foods, it may not make any difference, but some use chemicals routinely in their growth. Although they are slightly more expensive, consider this for your meal plans for the next 30 years. We are simply trying not to screw up your normal biome. Also, wash your fresh food off before preparation. I am not as concerned about bugs as I am about chemicals.

One last thing. I talked about carbs and protein, now about fats, specifically omega 6 and omega 3 fatty acids. Remember the difference is where the double bond is located. Historically it appears the ideal ratio of omega 6/omega 3 fatty acids in the diet was about 1-2/1. Now it is 16/1. The primary source of omega 6 in the diet is soybean oil. In 1900 the average intake of soybean oil per capita in the USA was about zero. In 2000 it is 24 pounds per person.

Again, is this just a coincidence or does this also have something to do with our unhealthy diet over the last 60 years? When we measure the amount of omega 6 fatty acids in our fat stores, we find this has increased 3X over the last 50 years. Omega 6 fatty acids are associated with promoting inflammation, Omega 3 with lowering inflammation. Progressively more diseases are being attributed to an abnormal inflammatory response.

I have not spoken about GMO products, but most soybean (and corn) are GMO products. Both are fed to animals to finish them, which means to feed them high-fat products in a feedlot the last few months before slaughter to put weight on the animals and increase their fat content. The fat content in these animals contains a higher ratio of Omega 6/Omega 3 fatty acids than does grass-fed beef. Now you may understand why your supermarket is suddenly selling beef labeled grass-fed. The same can be true for other livestock including chickens and eggs. You may want to start reading the fine print on these products. They are almost always more expensive.

Food engineer, please notice. Many believe we eat too much soybean in our diet. Start reading the ingredients in what you buy (also look for HFCS and sucrose). How about grass-fed. How about lower omega 6/omega 3 ratios? Much of this information is written right on the package. Make sure you bring your glasses as the print is small.

CHAPTER 18

FINISH ALREADY

You started out wanting to lose weight. I talked you into wanting to lose fat. To speak the lingo, we had to do a little learning. Finally, I got around to telling you what the ketogenic diet was and how to get you there. I tried to get you to understand this is a temporary fat losing diet and when you get to your goal, you must get another diet. Usually, it must be different than the diet that got you to the point that you needed to lose weight.

I admit it. I am trying to get you healthy, not just by losing weight, but by changing your entire lifestyle for perhaps the next 30 years. I have addressed the maintenance diet with general guidelines, particularly for a food engineer, which in most cases is going to be the wife/mother. I need to emphasize what an important and difficult job this is. In fact, it is quite difficult to do correctly unless this is a full-time job.

I talked about fasting and its benefits. It is a normal part of your body's homeostasis. Do not be afraid of fasting a little. I insist on the 12 hours nighttime fast as a minimum.

I ended with a few ideas that were slightly speculation. We all agree something has happened to us and our health over the last 60 years. I examined how our diet has changed since I believe this is the major cause of our problems. Although our health care has dramatically improved, almost to the performing miracles stage, our lifespan is not that much different than 2500 years ago. I have tried to discourage the thinking that anything worth knowing has come about in the last 50 years, to recognizing there were just as many if not more geniuses 4000 years ago as there are now, and we can't just throw away their ideas. New information may come up on some of my ideas and you will adapt your thinking accordingly. I have no special knowledge or ideas.

Food Engineers Only:

Get a diet you can stick with for everyone for a long time.

There are festive occasions. Just stay with the diet most of the time

About a third from each food group. A little less with carbs and a little more with fat

People eat until they are full. If someone wants to lose a little weight, skip eating a day. Then the next day go back to regular eating. Some may want to do this a couple of times a week, but even then, still eat normally on the eat days. We do not want a reduced calorie diet, but rather want to reset your weight set point.

Kids are different.

Within each food group make wise decisions:

Carbs: Decrease sucrose, does not have to be to zero

Stop HFCS. Get it close to zero.

Eat whole fruits. Some are better for you than others. Bananas are essentially dessert.

Figure out bread on your own. The best would be home-made with no preservatives.

Eat more vegetables.

Protein: Keep good gut health

Fats: Decrease soybean oil (check ingredients)

Low omega 6/omega 3 ratio.

Gut health: Organic foods, wash food, use your common sense. This includes avoiding unnecessary medication. This includes over the counter supplements.

Spend more money on food. Eat out less

12 hours fast daily. Maybe once a month skip a day eating.

If you and your friends find themselves in an emergency where there is no food available for a few days, I hope you will think this is no big deal if I do not eat 2-3 days, and don't panic and start eating your friends.

Finally, my favorite question: You are on a wagon train in the old west heading for Hollywood. You have two wagons when, during a thunderstorm, the horses run one of them off a cliff. You have four weeks to go but only half your food. Would you:

Have everyone eat half rations for four weeks.

Fast a week, full rations a week, fast a week, full rations a week.

What is the answer Grasshopper?

I have a reference book which is a combination of five other books called *Diet and Health* and contains further information on all the subjects covered in this book.

ADDENDUM I

<u>LIPOPROTEINS</u>

WARNING: Reading this chapter may cause drowsiness. Do not read while operating heavy equipment.

This field is changing all the time and even now, this information may be outdated. I revise this article at times, but even I cannot figure out what may be correct. Use this article as an approximation of what is really going one.

This is a chapter about lipoproteins. I have included this to give those on the ketogenic diet some information about their cholesterol level, as it may (or may not) increase slightly on the ketogenic diet. Nowadays, your insurance plan may provide a free comprehensive metabolic profile for you. Now you are going along feeling fine, and one of your lab tests is abnormal. Now you have opened a can of worms and the follow-up tests may not be free. Overall, this free test done on people who have no complaints, may be a boon to the insurance company and may not significantly help you. Cholesterol is one of these tests and, if you are not eating a low-fat diet, it may make it appear that your cholesterol level is too high, and you will get the statin prescription.

You might want to consider the risk/benefit ratio of taking this medication. I am going to include it here for the postgraduate food engineer for them to discuss this subject to those who may be asking them what they are doing. This subject is changing all the time and even during my brief lifetime, I have discovered what I thought I knew about this was incorrect or incomplete and have had to learn something new. I am warning you, next year I may have to retract this information and force you to but a new edition of the book. This chapter has been written in some of my other books.

Let me talk more specifically about T2DM and lipoproteins. There is an ongoing discussion about statin usage. Statins lower your cholesterol level. It appears that if you at high risk for cardiovascular disease, such as having had a heart attack or stroke, your survival will be improved if you take statins. It may or may not be causally related to the cholesterol lowering effect of statins, but never-the-less; even I must agree the effect is there. Therefore, if you are at a high risk of cardiovascular disease, statins may help you. Keep in mind you don't get something for nothing and there are side effects of statins, but in general, the benefit outweighs the risk.

Now if you have T2DM, you may be put in the high-risk category. By the time you have the T2DM diagnosis, several things have already gone wrong with your metabolism and even changing your diet may not be enough to correct things. Therefore, I give up and you may need statins for secondary prevention. Remember the purpose of my book is the common maintenance diet, and I am trying to prevent you from getting diabetes to start with.

Things are a little different if you just have obesity or prediabetes. You may or may not be in a high enough risk category such that statins will help you live longer. You and your health care provider need to figure that out. One of the side effects of statins is that it may increase your risk of developing diabetes. I am not sure if that will happen if you agree with the book, even if you decide to go on statins.

If you do not have heart disease and you take statins for five years, we must treat 104 people to prevent one additional heart attack. We must treat 154 people to prevent one additional stroke. Many believe the side effects of statins are underestimated.

It turns out that now health insurance offers a free screening physical every year. Included in the physical is some lab work. Part of this lab work may be cholesterol screening. If you are on the ketogenic diet, you eat low carbs and hence high fat. Usually, the percent of fat in your ketogenic diet is higher than that of protein. If your total cholesterol goes up, your health care provider may tell you to get off that crazy diet and go back to the high carbohydrate diet which made you go on the ketogenic diet in the first place. Over the years, cholesterol testing has evolved from being a number to being divided into many segments to now being divided into smaller segments. Also, throughout the years, I have been having trouble staying awake while someone explains it to me; nevertheless, I will attempt to explain cholesterol in the diet without putting you to sleep.

Sixty years ago, we decided we had an epidemic of heart disease. It used to be people died of infectious diseases but, with the advent of antibiotics and vaccines, public health projects, now they were dying of heart disease. Doctors like to call things epidemics. It used to be they were real epidemics like the Spanish flu or the Black Plague, now they are heart disease or drug abuse or global warming. Epidemics sound dramatic. Anyway, when we investigated people who were dying of heart disease, we discovered they had plaques, called atheromas, clogging up their arteries. These plaques were made up of cholesterol. To fix this we had to reduce the cholesterol in our diet. This meant a low-fat diet which meant a high carb diet. Of course, no proof lowering cholesterol would work, but it's only common sense, isn't it?

The government got involved and for the last sixty years, we have been advised that we need to eat less fat. Billions of dollars have been spent to study this concept and billions spent advising people to cut down on fat eating. Despite all the studies, it is difficult to show either that the cholesterol level predicts heart disease or that lowering the cholesterol lowers heart disease. What we have done is made millions of people obese and drastically increased T2DM along with many other associated diseases. Even today, many health care providers believe a low fat (and high carb) diet is the best and exercise will help you lose weight, despite now a large body of evidence indicates otherwise.

At the beginning of the 20th century, several reports had come from Africa about the health and nutrition of native people. These were well documented through the British Foreign service and medical missionaries. The story was always the same. No diabetes, rare cancer, no GI disease, and no obesity until the western diet with processed food such as sugar and flour were introduced. After a few years, the Africans looked like modern Americans.

This was true despite what diet they were on before. Some were high fat, some low fat and high carbs. This story was repeated no matter what ethnic group was observed or what continent. This data was conveniently ignored. Science has progressed and now we have a better idea of what is going on and that is what I am going to try to explain. These same observations were made in North America with the American Indians.

Your body likes cholesterol and uses it for all kinds of things. Your brain is mainly cholesterol. Most of the cholesterol in your body you have made yourself. Cholesterol is a type of fat. You eat some fat in the form of triglyceride, the GI tract breaks down this fat into fatty acids, then the GI tract absorbs these fatty acids, and turns them back into triglycerides. It then binds these triglycerides together in a package formed with a protein called apolipoprotein B and phospholipids. This package gets dumped into the lymphatic system and eventually into the blood, bypassing the liver, unlike all the other nutrients that get absorbed. These packets are called chylomicrons.

We have five different categories of lipoproteins. Lipoproteins allow fat to be transported in the blood. Fat does not dissolve in water, so you must use something like soap to get it suspended. The fat in your blood needs to be suspended otherwise it would just all float to the top. Lipoproteins perform this function and thus distribute the fat around your body to be used by the cells for energy and to make things. The lipoproteins are all less dense than water since they contain fat. To separate them we use a centrifuge and so we named them from the least dense to the densest. The least dense have the largest fat component.

Chylomicrons: Made in the gut. No cholesterol. Lots of triglycerides and thus least dense

VLDL: Very low-density lipoproteins. These are made in the liver. Contain some cholesterol

IDL: Intermediate density lipoproteins. These come from VLDLs. Contain more cholesterol

LDL: Low-density lipoproteins. Divided into two subsets of small dense LDL (sdLDL) and large buoyant LDL, (lbLDL) which are sometimes known as large fluffy LDL

HDL: High-density Lipoproteins. These can uptake cholesterol in the tissues as well as transfer cholesterol and apos to other particles

OK, I am starting to get sleepy. I'm sure you are too. If you want, you can skip to the last paragraph to see how this applies to you. If not, I am going to rest a while then continue. You nerds are welcome to follow along.

The chylomicrons get in the blood and interact with HDL to obtain different types of apolipoproteins, which allow them to bind to cell receptors and activate the enzyme which breaks down triglyceride into fatty acid. The fatty acid is absorbed by the cell, and the chylomicron continues its journey to donate elsewhere.

Eventually, it runs out of triglyceride and goes back to the liver to be broken down and the components reused. So, when you eat fat, this is what happens. Notice the liver is not involved much till the end. Also, notice no glucose or fructose was used in this process to create any fat.

Next, we have the VLDL. These carriers of cholesterol and triglycerides originate in the liver where apoB is also made and turned into lipoprotein particles. Note that chylomicrons are composed of triglycerides that you eat, while VLDL is composed of triglycerides that the liver has made from excess glucose and fructose. When you eat sucrose, the glucose portion goes into the blood and used for energy by the body. The fat cells take up some of the glucose under the influence of insulin and make triglycerides for storage. The liver can also take up some of the excess glucose and make triglycerides.

As for the fructose part of the sucrose, the liver does not dump it into the bloodstream, although at high doses some does leak into the blood. Most is processed into glycogen or made into triglycerides. Most of your triglycerides made in the liver come from fructose; fructose in sucrose, HFCS, and also some from actual fruit. When your liver makes triglycerides, it also must make a particle to transfer the triglyceride in the blood. This particle is VLDL; hence, the more fructose, the more triglyceride, the more apoB particles. The VLDL particle circulates in the blood and picks up a few slightly different apolipoprotein proteins in addition to interacting with HDL lipoprotein particles which donate some apoE proteins.

You can see how this can make you sleepy. There are numerous apoB particles that are slightly different. When I say apoB, I mean apoB100. There are also apoC and apoE particles, but the exact name is not important, just the general story as to what is happening.

Anyway, after the VLDL picks up some additional apoproteins, it becomes mature and proceeds on its journey to give up the triglycerides to various cells in the body by the activation of the lipoprotein lipase enzyme in the cell, and eventually becomes smaller and denser. There is a protein found in the blood called cholesterol ester transfer protein (CETP) which also collects some of these triglycerides in exchange for cholesterol from HDL lipoprotein particles. Hence as the VLDL loses triglycerides and gains cholesterol (which is denser), it becomes heavier and finally, we call it IDL.

The CETP protein and enzymatic process is one in which the lipoproteins gain cholesterol as they travel in the blood. They get progressively denser as they give up triglycerides and gain cholesterol. The triglycerides they gave up are used for energy and building things out of fatty acids. The cholesterol is used for building things like cell membranes or hormones.

We have chylomicrons, VLDL, and now IDL. All along we are getting denser particles. About half the IDL particles are taken up by the liver cells and broken down into their component parts, the other half continues to lose triglycerides and gain cholesterol and thus become denser and turn into LDL particles. One of the differences between IDL and LDL particles is the number of apoE proteins they contain. ApoE allows the lipoprotein particle to bind to the LDL receptors on the cell. When the IDL is converted into LDL, the apoE leaves and only the apoB is left. The affinity of the lipoprotein particle to the cell is then not nearly as much.

We started with triglycerides. The cells need it for energy (fatty acids) and cholesterol to build things in the cell. When the cell needs to build things out of cholesterol, it usually just makes the cholesterol. If it needs more, it makes receptors on the outside of the cell to bind LDL particles. It then engulfs these particles and uses the cholesterol or triglyceride.

One way it can regulate how many LDL particles it needs is to recycle the receptors or just digest them. LDL is not 'bad cholesterol" but is needed to transport cholesterol to be used by the cells. When we measure cholesterol in your blood, we measure all the cholesterol bound up in all the different lipoprotein particles.

Turns out just measuring all the cholesterol is not a very good predictor of heart disease. In fact, elevated HDL seemed to decrease your risk of heart disease. Since most of the cholesterol is transported in the LDL particles, we figured maybe if we just measured the LDL cholesterol it would be a better predictor. Turns out it worked a little better but not much. Half the people with heart attacks did not have elevated LDL. So, what's the deal?

As technology advanced, we were able to measure the LDL better. Since each LDL particle contains one apoB protein, we can count the number of particles of LDL. Turns out there are two divisions of

LDL to be made. One that is a smaller, denser particle, the other is a larger fluffier and less dense particle. The number of smaller dense LDL particles appears to be the best predictor of your risk of heart disease; therefore, the lower the number of sdLDL, the better.

Now let's see how we can figure out how to get fewer particles. If we eat fat, it appears in the blood as a chylomicron which does not contain any cholesterol. Remember we thought the atheroma made from cholesterol was the whole reason we started down this low fat/high carbohydrate diet pathway. Now it looks like eating fat had nothing to do with it.

What did cause this increase in lipoprotein particles? The liver had to make lots of VLDL (which eventually turns into LDL) to transfer all the extra triglyceride it was making from all the extra fructose, stimulated by the elevation of insulin, as a result of insulin resistance, as a result of high carbohydrate diets and processed food, which overwhelmed the liver's capacity to deal with carbohydrate intake. Do you mean to tell me we have been told to do the exact opposite of what we should have been doing?

First, let us finish up with HDL. These are manufactured in the liver with the main apolipoprotein being apoA. These are small dense particles (smaller than LDL) that can remove fat particles from cells and transport them for disposal. These include cholesterol, phospholipids, and triglycerides. We have already seen how it can trade cholesterol for triglycerides or transfer apoproteins to various other lipoprotein particles.

Let me insert this. Apolipoprotein A1 (apoA) is the major protein component of HDL particles. This protein accepts fats from with cells, including macrophages in the walls of the arteries, to transport elsewhere, including getting rid of them. It turns out that the ratio of apoB-100/apoA1 may have a stronger correlation with MI event rates than the other methods. The lower the better. This may be a refinement of the LDL/HDL ratio. We want more HDL, and less LDL.

Increasing concentrations of HDL are associated with decreasing accumulation of atherosclerosis within arterial walls. HDL can also transport out particles in atheromas, those plaques that clog up the artery. Usually, heart attack and stroke are more related to the rupture of these atheromas precipitating a clot rather than the progressive narrowing of the artery.

Back to LDL. The small particles appear to be more dangerous as they are small enough to penetrate the walls of the blood vessels. Once there, they are more likely to become oxidized. Oxidation changes the structure of the protein and fats in the particle and upsets the normal metabolism, also it damages the receptors. This also leads to an inflammatory reaction in which the macrophage cells engulf these cholesterol-containing particles and become laden with fat to become what are called foam cells. These make up the atheroma and induce inflammation.

The HDL particles are even smaller than the small LDL particles and can penetrate these areas to remove cholesterol.

Welcome back those of you who wisely decided to skip the nerd section. Now we know that total cholesterol levels do not predict heart disease. We also know that total LDL cholesterol does not predict heart disease very well. We do know that the number of small dense LDL particles does predict heart disease. We know there is another large fluffy LDL particle that does not appear to be associated with heart disease. We can test for the number of sdLDL particles, and we want there to be less. We also know that HDL particles can transport unwanted cholesterol out of the cell and perhaps out of atheromas, so we want more of them.

You went to the doctor. He said stop that ketogenic diet because it is raising your cholesterol and go back on the low-fat diet. He does not know that saturated fats increase the amount of HDL and increases the amount of large fluffy LDL, thus may decrease cardiovascular risk. He does not know that a high carbohydrate diet increases insulin and insulin resistance. He does not know that fructose is the main source of triglyceride that is made in the liver as a result of increased fructose consumption from sucrose, HFCS, and fruit. The liver must make particles to carry away this increased triglyceride load, so it makes more VLDL particles.

These eventually become LDL, and some become sdLDL particles, whose numbers are related to the increased triglyceride production by the liver. If the liver does not have an excess of triglycerides (low carb/fructose diet), the VLDL particles it produces become the large fluffy kind. If the liver is producing lots of triglycerides from excess fructose, the VLDL particles become the small dense kind.

In any case, the saturated fats in your diet have nothing to do with it. They are carried by chylomicrons which do not contain any cholesterol and are recycled by the liver when they have given up their loads. This is unlike the triglycerides made in the liver which are transported in VLDL particles and eventually become the sdLDL particles.

I will repeat the bottom line. In history, it appears as if a higher carb diet was eaten during times of lower food availability as these could be readily preserved. This calorie restriction seemed to protect somewhat against the elevated insulin and insulin resistance seen in modern high carb diets, which are eaten when there is still plenty of food available. Processed food like sucrose and flour leads to a more rapid absorption of glucose and fructose, which leads to an initial greater surge of insulin and more total insulin secreted. Repeat this several times a day for 20-30 years and you get insulin resistance with chronic high levels of insulin.

In addition, the heavy burden and rapid absorption of fructose lead to increased production of triglycerides in the liver, increased small dense LDL, and increased blood vessel disease. It also overwhelms the liver's ability to cope with the rapidly rising level, and thus increased fructose in the blood. Increased fructose and glucose lead to increased AGEs. Increased insulin leads to decreased insulin-degrading enzyme in the brain and hence decreased amyloid metabolism. Low saturated fat in the diet means high carbohydrates in the diet.

The absorption of saturated fats by the GI tract does not increase the number of VLDL particles produced by the liver. Increased triglyceride production from excess fructose and glucose does increase the number of particles produced. It appears saturated fats increase total cholesterol by increasing HDL and large fluffy LDL, something we want to happen. Eating several times a day and never fasting, decreases autophagy.

If you recall the chapters on AGEs and autophagy, you know increased AGE production results in crosslinking of proteins and stiffness in the arterioles. These AGEs cannot be easily removed and contribute to the actual aging of tissues. The goal is to prevent their generation, which has been increased by our high carbohydrate consumption, which has been dictated by a low-fat consumption. Lower fat in the diet means higher carbs.

As I have told you before, the human body is extremely complex. I am giving you approximately what is going on; enough for you to make some informed decisions. We discover different particles all the time and try to incorporate them into the discussion of lipoproteins. I have tried to give you enough knowledge that you can halfway understand what the scientists are telling you and use your common senses. Essentially, I am teaching you some of their lingo.

I hope you can use the information here to make some reasonable decisions regarding your diet and what food you buy and eat.

Remember, these scientists are the same people who told you to eat a low-fat diet for 75 years. Now they think maybe that wasn't a great idea.

This addendum has been published on its own in an eBook and as an audiotape. Also present on the website, kellygregg.com, as a podcast.

ADDENDUM II

<u>DIETS SHORT VERSION</u>

Believe it or not, some are calling the people crazy who are on the ketogenic diet. Here is the Cliff note version to show your friends.

Eat no more than 25 grams of absorbable carbohydrates daily. Eat as much fat and protein as you want. Eat until your hunger is satisfied. You do not need to eat any vegetables or fruit unless you can squeeze it into the 25 grams of carbs.

Best historical diet: Eat when you are hungry and stop when you are full. This also turns out to be the usual diet for most people and it has seemed to work fine for most of history. In modern times, many became overweight following this diet. We used to explain this by saying you just gain weight when you get older because you don't exercise as much. Some people exercise a lot, some not so much. The amount of exercise makes little difference, but more to the point is why some people don't exercise much. Is it possible that despite being fat, they do not have enough energy? Some say it's just genetics.

If you believe in evolution, do you think that somehow this is an evolutionary advantage? How come we just got fat for the last few hundred years? I believe the diet over the last couple hundred years is the problem, not some worldwide cellular mutation.

Weight loss diets:

Fasting: Best weight loss diet. you can only do this if you have fat. Hunger down. Energy up. Not a maintenance diet

Ketogenic diet: 25 grams carbs. Eat till satisfied. Hunger down. Energy up. Not a maintenance diet

Normal diet and exercise. It does not usually work to lose weight. In fact, we would expect you to gain weight through increased muscle mass. Poor fat losing diet. If this is the usual American diet, eventually you may end up with more muscle but fatter than when you started. Hunger up. Energy down. Not enough fatty acid production by the fat cells to supply cellular energy needs; hence, your body must lower the metabolic rate. Still carbs present to increase insulin which forces more energy into fat cells.

Reduced calorie diet: Hunger up. Energy down. You tend to gain weight after you eventually quit the diet. Hardly anyone can stay on this for long. Not many fatty acids for energy; hence, the body may need to lower the metabolic rate to maintain energy balance. (You do get some increase in fatty acids production for energy, just not nearly as much as the keto diet; and your hunger will eventually drive you to fail the diet.

Reduced calorie diet with exercise: Even more hunger.

Ketogenic with exercise: Does not increase hunger. More fat loss than plain keto, less than fasting. Weight goes down; remember you may also gain muscle mass. That is not necessarily a bad thing unless you get crazy about it. As your energy demand goes up, more fatty acids and ketones are provided. No need for the body to make any metabolic rate adjustments. Low insulin levels keep glucose and fatty acids from being absorbed into the fat cells and allow more energy available for the rest of the cells in the body. An elevated protein and fat diet also appears to suppress hunger, so in addition to increasing your fatty acid production from fat, you may be not eating quite as much as you are not as hungry.

These are all temporary weight-loss diets. On the keto diet, you do not have to eat many vegetables or fruit. You will not get any nutritional disease. If that scares you, go down and buy some cheap multivitamins that contain Vitamin C. Remember, the Inuit culture in the past (today they eat normal junk food). They hardly ever ate a vegetable or fruit, yet they still were healthy.

This is my best current idea as to what happened. In the past, people ate when hungry. Sometimes it was a carb-heavy diet, sometimes fat heavy. It seemed to be that there was a low rate of obesity. People did not get fat as they aged because they exercised less, they just naturally ate less as they followed their hunger.

You get hungry when your body needs energy. During keto and fasting, you are putting out plenty of fatty acids and ketones for energy. Insulin levels are low so there is a lower rate of fatty acids being absorbed by fat cells. Plenty of energy means decreased hunger. This is what should happen. You exercise more and get hungrier. If you did not exercise, then you did not get as hungry, and you did not eat as much. Your weight remained the same as your hunger managed the energy requirements.

In previously studied cultures, obesity became a problem when the western diet which had more carbohydrates. Appeared. The normal mechanism went awry and there was more hunger. People still ate when they were hungry, but as the energy input increased, eventually fat increased. If people just would not eat as much, they would not get fat, but apparently, something in the carbohydrates made them hungry. We kind of know now that this was a result of increased processed carbs in the western diet which caused faster absorption , which meant increased insulin. If the insulin level was high for a long enough time, we got insulin resistance and constant higher levels. When insulin is up, energy is being put into fat cells as glucose is being absorbed and changed into fatty acids. This lowers the energy available to the other cells and thus induces hunger.

You get fat because you eat more because you are hungry. As you can see, if you had a lot of fat cells and high insulin, you would be taking a lot of the energy out of the blood by it being forced into and the fat cells, thus increasing hunger. A vicious cycle, more fat cells, more cells to absorb energy under insulin influence, less energy available to cells, stimulation of hunger to increase energy intake until homeostasis has been restored.

A lean person does not have as much fat and hence cannot remove energy from the blood as well as a fat person; not only because the insulin is lower, but also because there are fewer fat cells. Therefore, a fat person is hungrier. This may be true even though the fat person is using up more energy just moving that weight around. Eventually, the body reaches a stable position so that the energy available to the cells is at a homeostatic level.

A fat person eats energy, enough that it should provide the cells all the energy they need. Some of this energy is abnormally taken up by the fat cells under the influence of insulin and stored. Now there is not enough energy to go around, and the fat person is hungry.

A lean person has a lower insulin level. The same amount of energy eaten now is enough for the cells and hunger is gone. If too much energy is taken in, the body simply increases the metabolism to match the intake. You could overcome this regulatory mechanism by forcing yourself to eat when you were not hungry, but this is difficult to do. Of course, if you continually eat a high carbohydrate diet as part of a diet that supplies sufficient energy, you end up with insulin resistance and back to the previous paragraph.

If the metabolism was normal, then if you ate more, hunger went down, and energy went up. If you did not have enough energy, hunger went up. Nobody got fat.

I have become convinced that it is not just that carbs are available in our modern diet, but that processed food may be the main culprit. Sucrose, HFCS, fruit juices, finely ground wheat flour: all promote rapid absorption of carbohydrates as we previously discussed. This may be the main driver of insulin resistance. One cup apple juice is 4 apples and contains 26 grams of carb. It takes five minutes to drink. Four apples take twenty minutes or longer to eat. Juice absorbed rapidly. Four apples absorbed over about 60 minutes. (this is an estimate). Which do you think would stimulate insulin the most? Fruit juice is a processed food.

Hunger is the main controller of energy input. Insulin resistance increases hunger. Low insulin decreases hunger. A low carb diet will eventually decrease hunger. This may be one of the reasons it works. As long as you don't force yourself to eat when not hungry, you will eventually lose enough fat to achieve your normal weight. This is where genetics comes into play as some people are thin no matter what, and some are husky. Nobody is fat unless something abnormal happens. Some people may be more sensitive to elevated carbohydrates and processed food than others, but they still should respond to the low carb/low processed food diet.

Eventually, go on the maintenance diet.

I edit and revise these books every six month to a year. As time has gone on, I am more impressed by the role of the gut biome in obesity and diabetes. Many studies have shown that a diabetic gut biome is different from a non-diabetic biome. Why is that? I suspect it is mainly the diet.

I have also been impressed by the epigenetic changes in the gut biome based on diet. These occur much more rapidly than I previously thought. We get insulin resistance from our diet, but is the biome we get from the western diet (and modern environmental effects) an almost equal factor?

I will be writing a series of books similar to *the Diet and Health* which will address epigenetics in diet and health, as well as much more information on the gut biome in diet and health. Of course, to do that, I will have to teach you more about chromosomes, genes, and epigenetics.

Maybe next year.